Implanted and Injected Materials in Urology

Implanted and Injected Materials in Urology

Edited by

Jean Marie Buzelin

Professor, Clinique Urologique,
Place Alexis Ricordeau,
44035 Nantes, France

ISIS
MEDICAL
MEDIA

Oxford

British Library Cataloguing in Publication Data. A catalogue record for this title is available from the British Library

ISBN 1 899066 15 2

Buzelin J (Jean Marie)
Implanted and Injected Materials in Urology
Jean Marie Buzelin

Always refer to the manufacturer's Prescribing Information before prescribing drugs cited in this book.

Set by
Marksbury Typesetting Ltd, Midsomer Norton, Bath, UK

Printed by
Biddles Ltd, Guildford & Kings Lynn, UK

Distributed by
Times Mirror International Publishers, Customer Service Centre, Unit 1,
3 Sheldon Way, Larkfield, Aylesford, Kent ME20 6SF UK

Contents

List of Contributors

David M. Barrett MD
Professor of Urology, Chair, Department of Urology, Mayo Clinic, 200 First Street SW, Rochester, MN 55905, USA

Luigi Cormio MD
Chair of Urology 'R', University of Bari, Policlinico, 70 124 Bari, Italy

Mary G. Donovan MD
Department of Urology, Mayo Clinic, 200 First Street SW, Rochester, MN 55905, USA

Eduardo Kleer MD
Department of Urology, Mayo Clinic, 200 First Street SW, Rochester, MN 55905, USA

Bo-Johan Norlén MD
Department of Urology, Akademiska Sjukhuset, Uppsala University, 751 85 Uppsala, Sweden

Denis C. O'Sullivan MD
Department of Urology, Royal Liverpool Hospital, Prescot Street, Liverpool L1 8XP, UK

Bhalchandra G. Parulkar MD
University of Massachusetts Medical Center, 55 Lake Avenue North, Worcester, MA 01655, USA

Mirja L. Ruutu MD PhD
Consultant in Urology, Department of Surgery, Helsinki University Central Hospital, 00290 Helsinki, Finland

Claude C. Schulman MD
Professor of Urology and Chief, Department of Urology, University Clinics of Brussels, Erasme Hospital, 808 route de Lennik, B-1070 Brussels, Belgium

Martti Talja MD PhD
Consultant in Urology, Department of Surgery, Päijät-Hämeen Central Hospital, 15850 Lahti, Finland

Gordon Williams MS FRCS
Department of Surgery, Hammersmith Hospital, Du Cane Road, London W12 0HS, UK

Preface

The use of injected and implanted materials will be a challenge for urologists in the coming years, even if the problem of biocompatibility is still not completely solved. Non-autologous materials are likely to cause granulomas at the injection site, and also tend to migrate. The risk of migration is thought to be inversely proportional to the particle size, and, consequently, slight with the recent non-autologous materials. Autologous materials such as fat and collagen are better in terms of biocompatibility, but they carry the risk of resorption and thus the clinical effects may not last.

The principle of endoscopic correction of vesico-ureteral reflux is to create a solid support behind the intravesical ureter by endoscopic injection of materials, thereby elongating the intramural length of the ureter. The injection technique is simple and can be performed as a day-case procedure. Procedure-related complications are rare, and the short hospitalization time significantly reduces the peri- and post-operative pain. The most recent studies indicate an overall success rate higher than 90%, reaching 65% after the first injection. However, the use of non-autologous injectable substances for the treatment of vesico-ureteral reflux is still debated; disadvantages include particle migration, with subsequent volume loss at the injection site, granuloma formation, and possible latent carcinogenic effects. In fact, the only significant complication with the endoscopic procedure remains the failure to abolish reflux at the initial injection.

Urinary incontinence is a common and often neglected condition, which treatment should be offered in a stepwise fashion beginning with the least invasive therapy. Among non-invasive procedures, injected materials (polytef, collagen, autologous fat, silicone) can be offered as a relatively simple day case procedure and has potential not only as an effective treatment option but also in reducing the cost for treating incontinence. The best candidates for treatment with injectable materials are those with intrinsic sphincter deficiency with good anatomical support and urodynamic or radiological evidence of failure of the proximal part of the urethra to close at rest in the absence of detrusor contraction. It offers an attractive alternative to surgery especially in the elderly and those unfit for major surgery.

There is a range of implantable stents available with differing characteristics: coefficient of friction, tensile strength, memory, internal-external diameter ratio and chemical inertness. They also have deleterious effects upon the urothelium, including encrustation, stone formation, bacterial adherence, and infection. It was suggested as well that ureteral stents have an obstructive effect, with urinary drainage being around rather than through the stent lumen, unless pressures are very high. Noxious effects of reflux inside the stent are unimportant, although a significant decrease of the pelvic pressure following bladder drainage has been demonstrated in animal experiments. Other complications of stents include loin pain, migration and dysuria. It was contended that 'stents do more harm than good' unless the ureter is obstructed, or following endoscopic or open ureteric surgery.

In 1980 Fabian reported the use of a stainless steel coil as a stent in the prostatic urethra in patients who would otherwise have been treated with a long term urethral catheter. The finding that stents manufactured of a woven mesh of super-alloy, titanium, or nickel/titanium would become covered with normal urothelium, led to the introduction in 1987 of so-called permanently implanted stents. However it became clear that the insertion of a stent into the prostatic urethra resulted in severe dysuria, frequency and urgency in a significant proportion of the patients. Nowadays, permanently implanted stents for the treatment of prostatic obstruction should still be considered experimental. To reduce the incidence of these complications, modifications of the original stainless steel spiral have taken place and several new stents were introduced. These stents are referred to as temporary stents in that they are not incorporated into the urinary tract and can be easily removed. These have been used to treat prostatic obstruction, urethral strictures and neurological voiding disorders. They are considerably less expensive than a permanent stent and might be used as an alternative. In a review of published data, out of over 900 patients treated, approximately 70% of temporary prostatic stents achieved their objective, i.e. they remained *in situ* until the patient died with a functioning stent or underwent planned surgery.

In 1973, Scott introduced a totally implantable artificial urinary sphincter (AUS), the first one with a well defined urethral closure pressure. The evolution of the AUS has gone through several phases and has ultimately ended up at the AS 800. AUS works like a physiological sphincter providing continence without obstruction; this is obvious when comparing maximum urethral pressure while the AUS is inflated or deflated. So, AUS is only indicated in cases of incontinence due to sphincteric insufficiency. At first, it was used for treating intractable incontinence for which surgical procedures do not provide good results; namely neurogenic incontinence and incontinence succeeding prostatectomy. Nowadays, indications extend to recurrent female urinary stress incontinence. The outcome is excellent in male and female incontinence with a success rate higher than 90%. It is a little more disappointing in cases of congenital neuropathic bladder because in more than half of the patients, vesical compliance impairs several months after surgery. Unfortunately, complications are still not completely solved. Some lead to device explantation: erosion and sepsis. Some need a revisionary operation; for example, non-occlusive cuff, fluid leakage, tube kinking, pump dysfunction. In spite of these complications, the artificial urinary sphincter, is likely to be one of the most useful recent progresses in Urology.

The use of penile prostheses is more detectable. It is intended to provide penile rigidity upon demand in subjects who cannot initiate or maintain an erection sufficient for penetration. Moreover, the ideal implant must increase penile length and girth during intercourse, and allow the penis to return flaccid and non cumbersome otherwise. Many devices have been designed aiming to achieve this goal: rigid, semi-rigid, malleable and inflatable. But the more sophisticated they are, the more fragile and expansive they are too. Data about long-term safety and effectiveness are not available. In spite of the considerable number of implanted devices throughout the world, there are very few studies on patient and partner satisfaction. Most of the complications (infection, erosion, migration, extrusion, mechanical failures) have not been reported. The NIH Consensus Conference December 1992 recommended staging the treatment of erectile dysfunction, beginning with the less invasive ones such as pharmacotherapy, intracavernosal injection and vacuum device.

Total alloplastic replacement of the lower urinary tract will perhaps be an alternative to intestine bladder replacement. The ideal prosthetic bladder should be able to store a large amount of urine at a low pressure and to empty completely without reflux into the kidney. It would have volitional control. It would be made of a totally inert and biocompatible material. It would be surgically easy to implant and be accessible for repairs and replacement if needed. Such a prosthesis has never been implanted in a human being. The main cause of failure, in animal experiments, has been the development of fibrous capsule around the prosthesis restricting filling and emptying, leakage of urine at the urethral anastomosis, ureteric obstruction and encrustation leading to hydronephrosis. However solutions are in progress for overcoming these ultimate difficulties.

Jean Marie Buzelin

Biocompatibility of injected materials in urology

1

C. C. Schulman

Introduction

Non-autologous materials are widely used in the medical field today and also have a rich and illustrious past. Paraffin, petrolatum, vegetable oils, lanolin, beeswax, silicone, Teflon and collagen have all been injected into the human body as bulking agents for soft tissues.[1] These materials have been used in ENT, orthopaedics, gynaecology, plastic surgery and urology to name a few. The focus of this chapter is to emphasize the usage and biocompatibility of some well-known and other more recent non-autologous materials applied in urology.

Prosthetic materials that are administerable endoscopically must be biocompatible, non-toxic and permanent. The recent debate concerning experimental studies has focused on the quantity of the material injected, the site of injection, local reactions and potential migration to distant organs. It should be pointed out that more than a decade after the endoscopic correction of ureteral reflux was first proposed,[2] not a single case of clinical significance has been reported.

Migration

Despite encouraging success rates with the endoscopic treatment of urinary stress incontinence and vesico-ureteral reflux (see Chapter 2) most of the concerns have focused on both the biocompatibility of the foreign materials and the potential for migration. In particular the migratory potential of polytetrafluoroethylene (Polytef) has made paediatric urologists and paediatric surgeons cautious. The migration problem will be discussed for each of the three widely used injectable products: polytetrafluoroethylene (Polytef or Teflon), injectable collagen and particulate siloxane (Macroplastique).

Distant migration of Teflon particles to the pelvic lymph nodes, lungs, brain, kidneys and spleen of monkeys have been found 10.5 months after implantation in an experimental study.[3] Teflon particles within the injectable Teflon paste range in size from 4 to 100 μm, with more than 90% of the particles smaller than 40 μm (Fig. 1.1). In a follow-up study,[4] smaller injected volumes were placed suburetically in monkeys. Local migration around the bladder and distal migration to the periaortic and pelvic nodes and testicles in male monkeys was reported. Furthermore, it was found that the granulomas at the subureteric injection sites, monitored

1

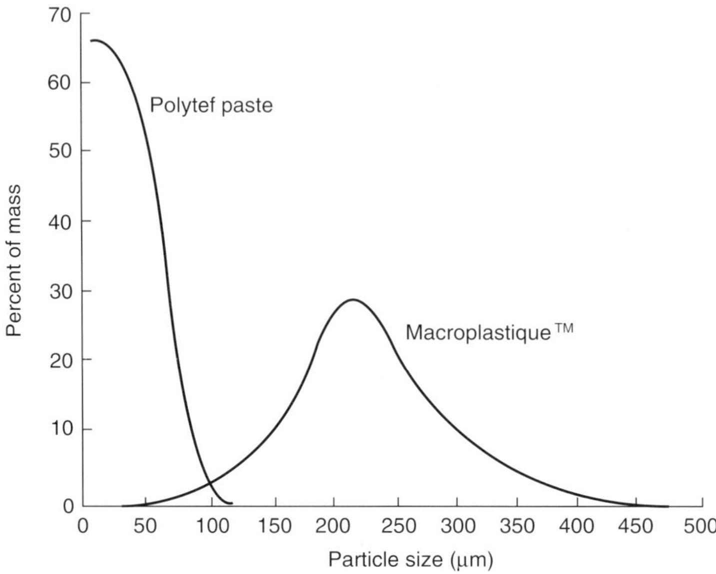

Fig. 1.1. Size distribution of Polytef paste particles[4] and Macroplastique[7] siloxane particles as measured by scanning electron microscopy. (Source: Malizia et al.[4] and Broutman Ltd.[7])

by CT scanning and MRI, enlarged over time and demonstrated persistent granulomas at autopsy.

Granuloma formations of Teflon particles that migrated to the lung in a patient that was treated with periurethral injections of large quantities of Teflon paste (total of two injections, one of which was up to 15 ml) have also been reported.[5] This is significant because it showed for the first time distant migration of Teflon particles to the lungs from an injection site in the urinary tract in humans. It should also be noted that 100 times more material was injected than would be expected for an endoscopic treatment of vesico-ureteral reflux. A second important fact from this case report is that although no measurements were given, using magnification scales provided by the authors, the three engulfed Polytef particles illustrated within the lung tissue measured 53, 42 and 37 µm (Table 1.1).

Migration itself is hypothesized to be dependent on the size of the foreign materials, with the critical size (80 µm) being that of the macrophages that can phagocytize them for transport to regional lymph nodes and possibly to distant organs.[6]

A particle-size analysis study[7] on Macroplastique indicates that the average particle size is 171 µm. A count reveals that 29% of the total number of particles range below 100 µm in diameter. However, 99.9% of the total volume of particles is made up of particles with diameters larger than 100 µm[7] (Fig. 1.1).

Migratory particles are engulfed along the perimeter of the injected materials. Smaller particles may in fact be located in the centre of the

Reference	Organ	Migration of particles
Monkeys and dogs		
Malizia *et al.*, 1984 [3]	Bladder and prostate	4–80 µm: Pelvic lymph nodes, lungs, brain, kidney and spleen
Malizia *et al.*,1988 [4]	Subureteric	Size? Periaortic and pelvic lymph nodes, testes
Humans		
Boedts *et al.*, 1967	Vocal cords	Up to 50 µm: Lymph nodes
Mittleman and Maraccini, 1983 [5]	Prostatic urethra	Up to 53 µm: Lung
Claes *et al.*, 1989 [16]	Periurethral	Largest ca. 40 µm: Lungs
Schulman *et al.*, 1990 [23]	Periureteral	Up to 50 µm: Lymph nodes

Table 1.1. Selected studies on Teflon migration

injected bolus surrounded by larger particles and not susceptible to distant migration. This has been shown for Teflon. Furthermore, because of the textured nature of the siloxane particles (Fig. 1.2) there is an increase in surface area and potential for 'anchoring' by host collagen (Fig. 1.3). Two recent studies[8,9] have shown very little migration of the large particled Macroplastique siloxane implants. The few particles that migrated were suggested as being the result of the injection technique, i.e. implanted extravesically. Collagen, on the other hand, is biodegradable and cited by various authors as being transient. Microscopically, bovine collagen forms numerous fine filaments rather than discrete particles, which upon injection form a compact mass at the injection site. However, there have been no experimental studies to indicate that this bundling would protect against further migration or degradation. A recent experimental study[10] notes that there are no distant granulomatous reactions found in tissues examined from various lymph nodes, liver, lungs and brain.

In the following section, the various non-autologous materials used for the correction of ureteral reflux will be described and discussed as to their biocompatibility.

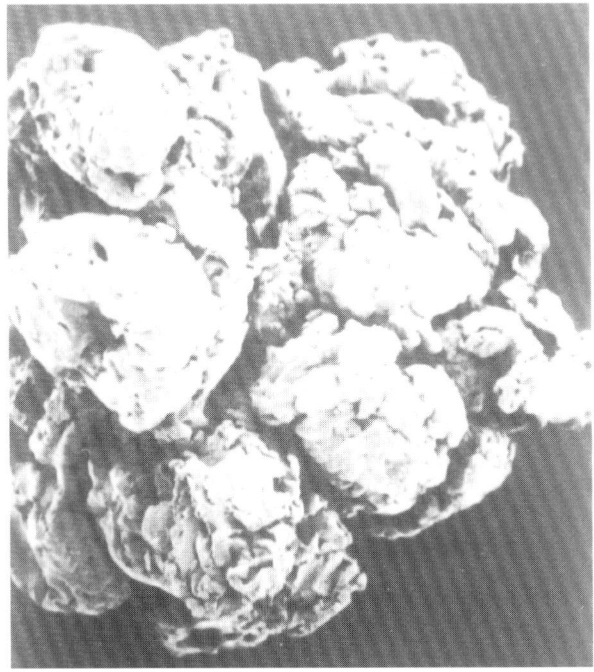

Fig. 1.2. Scanning electron microscopy of a micro-implant of Macroplastique. (Source: Beisang and Ersek[52]).

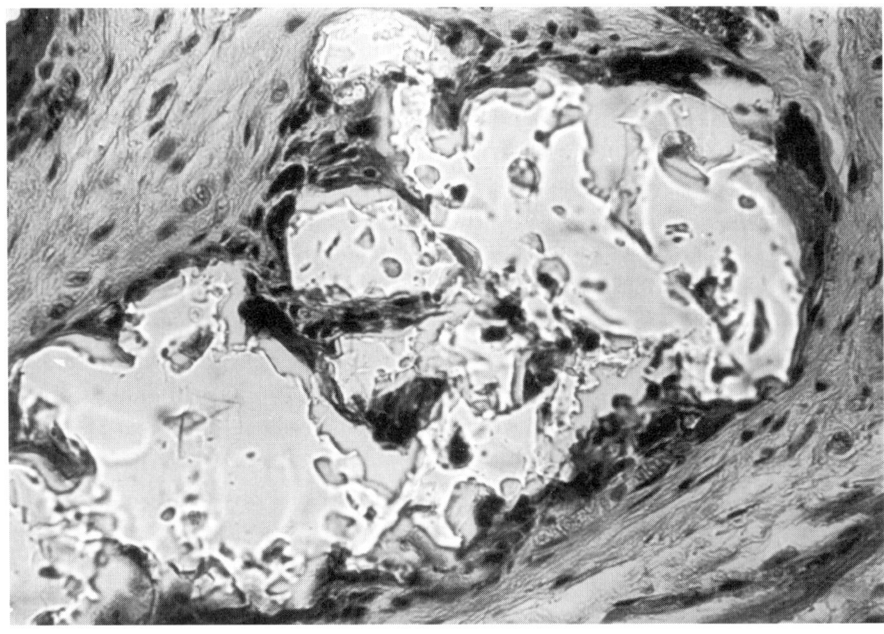

Fig. 1.3. High-power histological section showing strands of collagen that have been laid down by fibroblasts. Note that the micro-implants of Macroplastique are entirely encapsulated by collagen with some degree of ingrowth.

Injectable materials

Polytetrafluoroethylene/Teflon (Polytef)

Brand name: Urethrin

Commercially sold Urethrin consists of 33% polytetrafluoroethylene, 33% glycerine and 33% polysorbate. The polytetrafluoroethylene particles have an irregular surface and range from 4 to 100 µm in diameter, with more than 90% of the particles in the Teflon paste ranging from 4 to 40 µm in diameter[3] (Fig. 1.1).

Glycerine is used as lubricant but is also available as glyceryl trinitrate, a powerful vasodilator with a short action (20–30 min) and as glycerol suppositories, which maintain fluid levels in the large bowel by osmosis and vasodilation. The glycerine lubricant, because of its vasodilatory properties, is absorbed very quickly, probably taking the smaller particles of Teflon as well into lymphatic vessels. The remaining Teflon particles are usually encapsulated in their entirety with no collagen deposits between the individual particles (Fig. 1.4).

Injectable polytetrafluoroethylene (Polytef) has been used in many patients for vocal cord augmentation and for the management of urinary incontinence[11] since the early 1960s and 1970s, respectively. Non-injectable forms of Teflon have been used for sutures, hernia repair, replacement of the stapes, hip prostheses, cardiac valves and vascular grafts. Since 1984, many children have been treated with subureteric Polytef injection for the management of vesico-ureteric reflux.[12]

The treatment of young patients with Polytef remains problematic because of the reported potential of migration to distant organs and the potential of granuloma formation at the site of injection. Furthermore, questions have been raised as to possible carcinogenicity of this material, particularly in view of the fact that the substance may be within patients for decades. The available evidence does not confirm a significant carcinogenic effect in humans, rather, it suggests that, if there is a risk, it is extremely low.[13] This has been confirmed in rodents, where after long-term follow-up there was no evidence of epithelial or sarcomatous tumour formation.[14] However, human samples, taken decades after the implantation of Polytef, and long-term, non-rodent animal experiments are needed to substantiate the probable safety of Polytef in children. Some vociferous opponents propose the placement of a voluntary moratorium on the further use of Polytef for vesico-ureteral reflux.[15]

As mentioned above, migratory Teflon particles have been found in test animals in lungs, kidney, pancreas and brain tissue after injection in the bladder wall.[3,5,16,17,18] The migration is hypothesized to be due to the abundant presence of small particles with 90% of the Teflon particles measuring under 50 µm (see above).

(a)

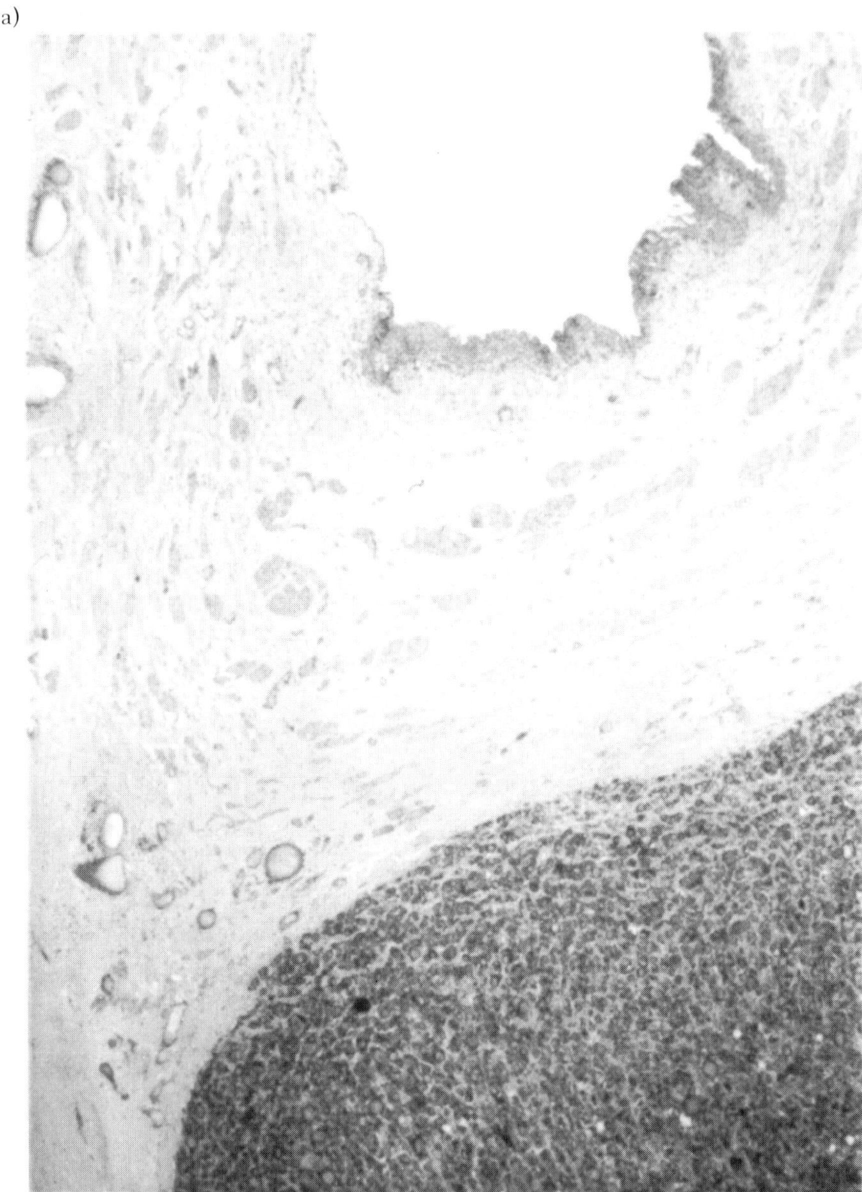

Fig. 1.4. (a) Teflon: granulomatous reaction at the site of injection. Individual Teflon spherules are not surrounded by collagen deposits.

Granulomas have also been reported after injection of Teflon.[3,5,16,19,20] A recent study[21] however doubts that reported migrated particles are in fact Teflon. Through X-ray micro-analysis and scanning electron microscopy no positive identification of Teflon particles could be made in distant organs of injected test animals. Rather, particles of sodium hypochlorite precipitate or reactive tissue products, which are morphologically indisting-

(b)

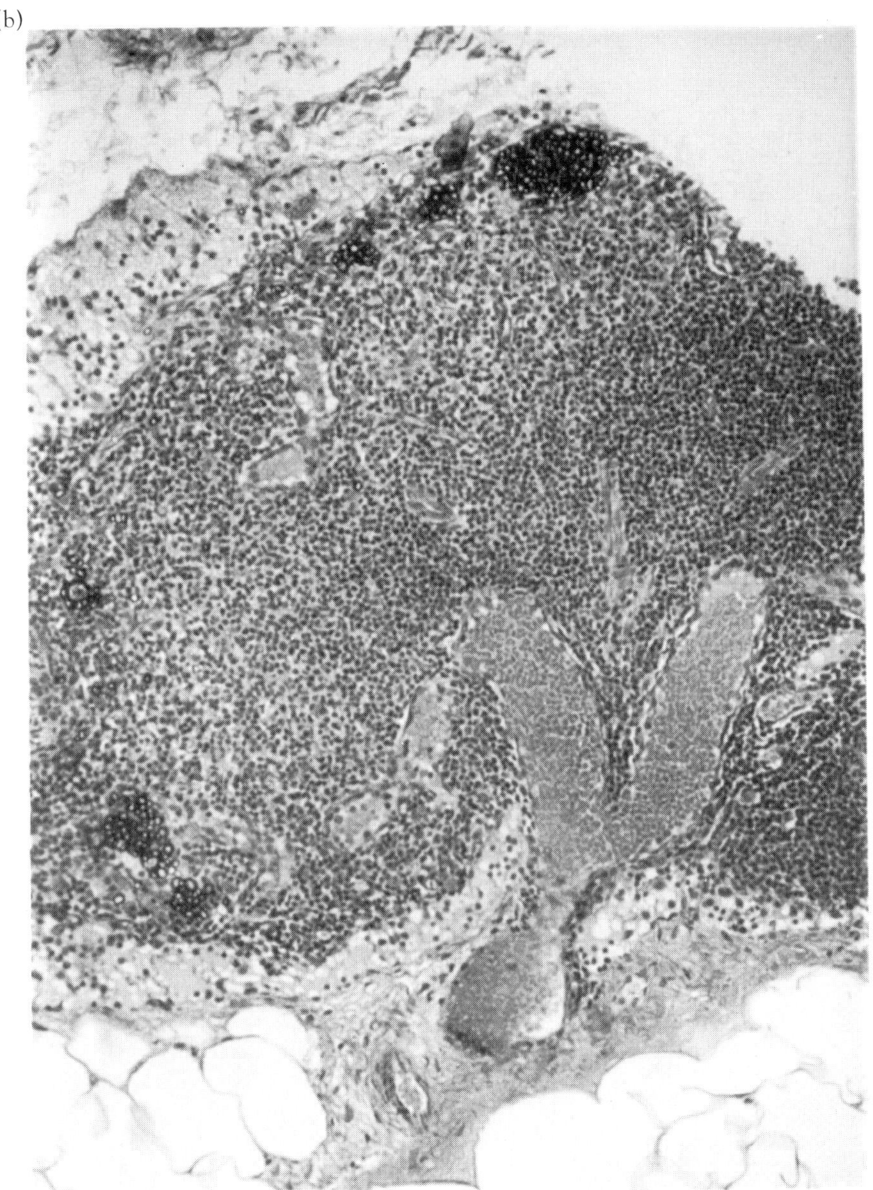

Fig. 1.4 (continued). (b) Teflon particle in lymph node.

uishable from polytetrafluoroethylene by polarizing light microscopy, have been hypothesized as being the structures in questions that researchers have been identifying as Teflon.

Nevertheless, the use of Teflon paste in cosmetic surgery for the treatment of wrinkles and furrows has, however, been abandoned because of severe chronic serious infections, whereas semi-solid Teflon implants (Gore-tex) are used.[22]

Histological findings of injected Polytef

Most histological findings of injected Teflon demonstrate local giant-cell granulomatous reaction at the injection site. The central portion of the Teflon granulomas are usually acellular and contain the largest quantity of Teflon. Macrophages with multinucleated giant cells containing Teflon spheres surround this area (Fig. 1.4).[10,23,24] Most studies report that the site and number of giant cells remained stable over time, in contrast to another study[25] showing that the lesions can be progressive over time.

Collagen, Gax-collagen and atelocollagen

Brand name: Gax-collagen; Contigen Implant

Contigen implant is composed of purified bovine dermal collagen that is lightly cross-linked with glutaraldehyde and dispersed in phosphate-buffered physiological saline. Atelocollagen is produced from bovine collagen by removing the telopeptide, which is the antigenic epitope of the collagen molecule (see below). Atelocollagen is therefore different from glutaraldehyde cross-linked collagen in terms of the way it excludes the epitope.

Collagen itself is the most abundant protein in the body and is in fact a term used for a variety of distinct fibrillar proteins, similar in structure.[26] The building blocks of these fibrillar proteins are called trimer collagen molecules consisting of three polypeptide chains (α-chains). Each α-chain contains approximately 1000 amino acids totalling up to 3000 Å (Fig. 1.5). Different types of α-chains have the same configuration but are distinct due to their composition and sequence of amino acids. However, they all have a glycine occupying the third position in the amino acid sequence. About 96% of the length of the chain is helical, with non-helical 'telopeptides' at the amino- and carboxyl-termini. These telopeptides contain the most important antigenic loci of the molecules, and play an important role in the association of α-chains determining the type of collagen molecule. Up to five types (types I–V) have been isolated.[1]

The purified injectable collagen is a suspension from 3.5% (used in urology) or 6.5% purified collagen derived from calf hide lightly cross-linked with glutaraldehyde dispersed in phosphate-buffered saline. The collagen itself is mainly type I collagen (95%), with traces of type III (5%). It has been made less antigenic by selective removal of the non-helical telopeptides. Other types of collagen are cross-linked with glutaraldehyde (Gax).

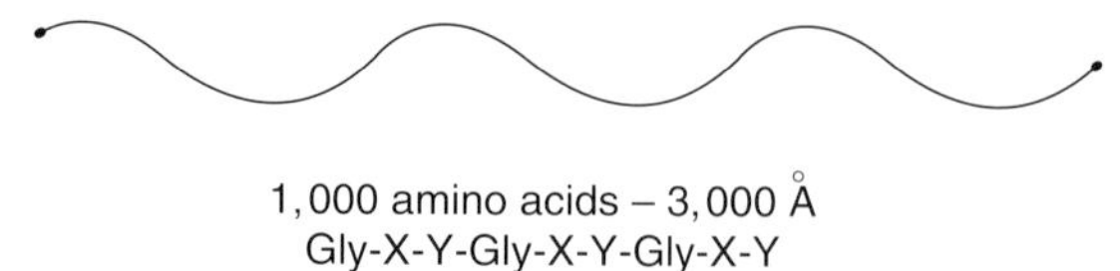

Fig. 1.5. Structure of the α-chain of collagen. (Courtesy Prof. G. Matton.)

Collagen is mainly synthesized by fibroblasts[26] and comprises an intracellular and extracellular phase (Fig. 1.6). Transcription of DNA occurs primarily at the long arm of chromosome 17 (type I collagen) and the long arm of chromosome 7 (types I and III) to form a messenger RNA. Translation occurs at the ribosomes of the rough endoplasmic reticulum. The formed polypeptide chain is a 'pro α-chain'. Three pro-α-chains form a three-dimensional helical procollagen molecule, with typical terminal telopeptides. After assemblage, the procollagen molecule is transported via the Golgi apparatus to the cell surface for release into the extracellular space. The telopeptides are then partially cleaved by specific peptidase and the collagen molecule is fashioned. Collagen molecules aggregate to form a collagen fibril which in turn cross-links to form a triple molecule. Further

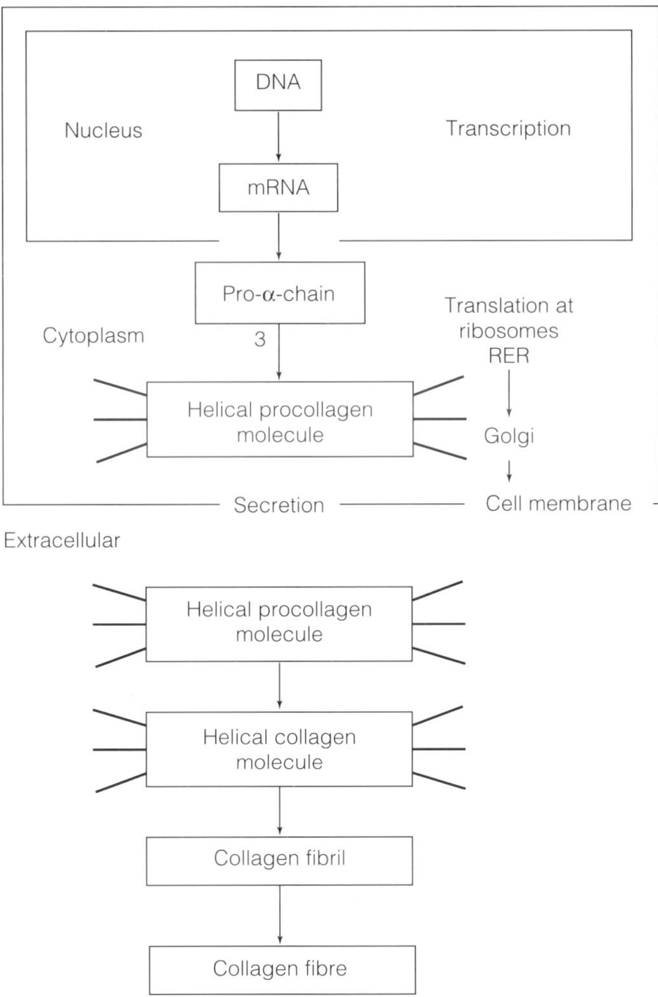

Fig. 1.6. Synthesis of collagen. (Courtesy Prof. G. Matton.)

cross-linking is possible between the α-chains of collagen fibres (Fig. 1.7).[27]

The breakdown of collagen is also very complex and will be briefly summarized here. Breakdown of collagen occurs by proteolytic attack by collagenases (synthesized by fibroblast, polymorphonuclear leukocytes and macrophages), capable of cleaving within the helical domain of the collagen molecule. The smaller collagen fragments are then proteolyzed by other proteases. The remaining fragments are then phagocytized and degraded by lysosomes.[1]

The glutaraldehyde cross-linking has a stabilizing effect on the collagen strands and slows down the digestion by the collagenases present within the macrophages which are drawn to the foreign bodies at the injection sites.[28]

Clinical results of injections with collagen from both human and bovine origin for the correction of soft-tissue contour defects were first published in 1977.[29] By 1984, the manufacturers of injectable collagen (Collagen Corporation) estimated that more than 100 000 patients had been treated.[30]

The use of Zyderm injections (injectable collagen brand name for plastic and cosmetic surgery and identical to the injectable collagen used for the endoscopic correction of reflux) has been widespread and enthusiastically applied by dermatologists and cosmetic surgeons beneath the wrinkles of millions of women and men for the past decade.

For the majority of plastic, cosmetic and dermatological surgeons, experience with collagen suspensions has been rather disappointing because the effect is of short duration (about one to three months).[31–34] Factors that have been cited affecting the duration and quality of the results are: (1) the technique of injection; (2) the location of implants (i.e. in a highly vascularized versus less-vascularized site); and (3) quantities used. This, therefore, also brings into serious doubt the ultimate fate of the injected collagen and the duration of the clinical results for correction of ureteral reflux and treatments of urinary stress incontinence in urology.

A recently presented experimental study[35] had as its aim a comparison between the behaviour of a second-generation collagen GAX 65 with the more commonly used GAX 35 (3.5% collagen by volume). GAX 65 is also a glutaraldehyde cross-linked bovine collagen, but with higher collagen concentrations (6.5% by volume). The invasion of fibroblasts into the implants and the formation of endogenous collagen types I and III was almost identical for both injectables. The main difference between the two products seem to be the better elevation properties and the better preservation of the volume of GAX 65.[35] No clinical results for urology of the latter have been presented.

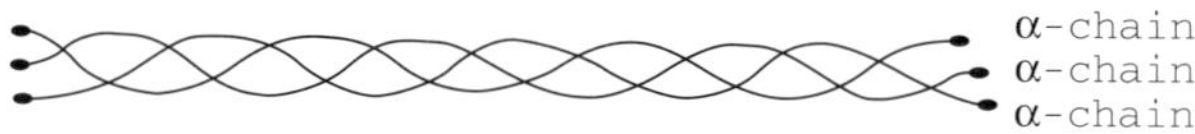

Fig. 1.7. Structure of the trimer collagen molecule. (Courtesy Prof. G. Matton.)

Because collagen is a foreign protein and potentially allergenic, skin testing is required several weeks before implantation. However, this does not always eliminate the danger of subsequent anaphylactic reactions.[36]

Histological findings of injected collagen

Injected collagen appears light pink with a haematoxylin/eosin stain and green in a Mason trichrome, and has a granular structure (Fig. 1.8). At two months, the collagen implant is surrounded by a fine fibrous tissue capsule, and fibroblast invasion begins from the periphery as a capillary ingrowth. The colonization by fibroblasts and subsequently fibrocytes towards the centre of the implant stabilized at nine months' follow-up (Fig. 1.9).[10]

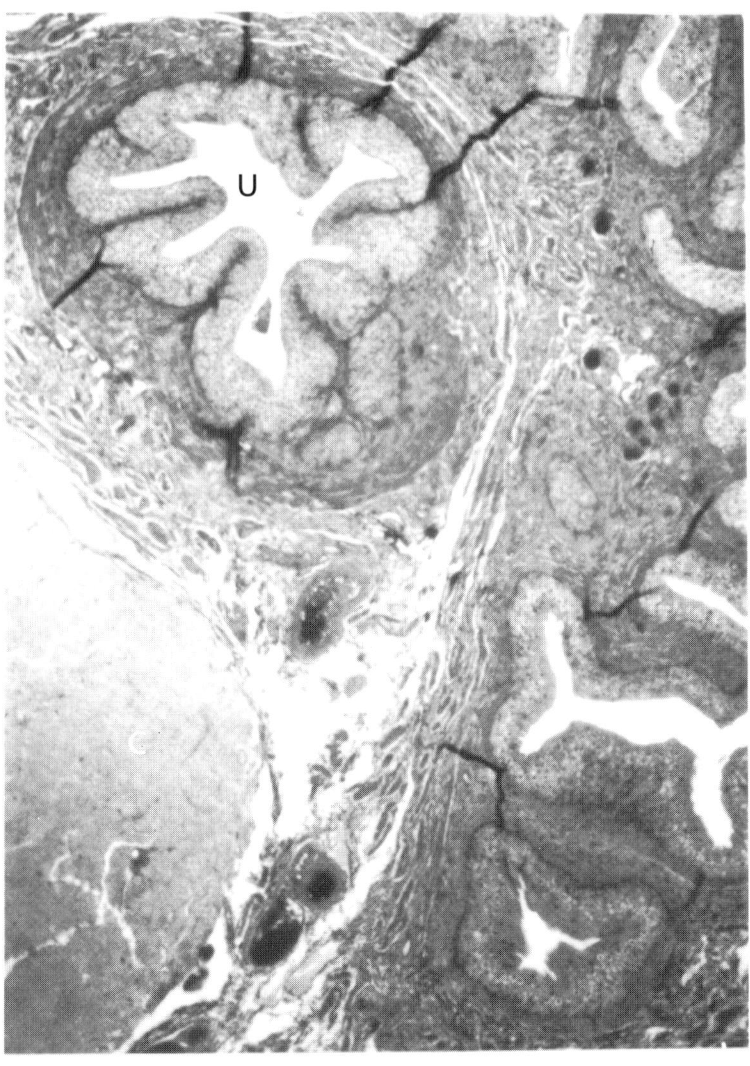

Fig. 1.8. Collagen (C) at the site of injection near the ureter (U).

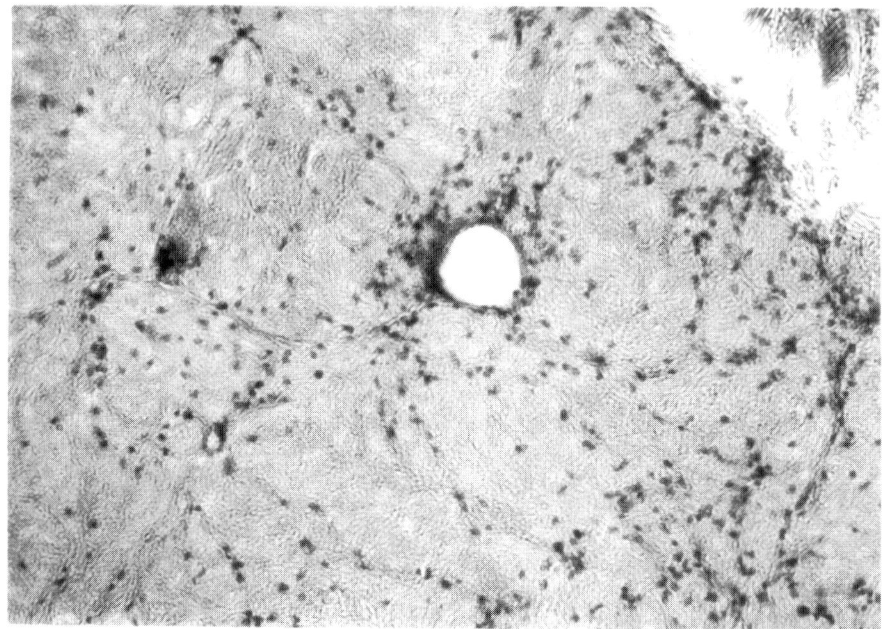

Fig. 1.9. Collagen colonization by fibroblasts.

There was no perifocal inflammatory reaction. This confirms earlier findings[37] indicating that in humans the glutaraldehyde cross-linked bovine collagen engendered a minimal localized inflammatory reaction without causing granuloma formation. Endogenous fibroblasts invade the bovine collagen implant and cells show active production of new human collagen, types I and III, replacing the initial implant.[17]

Polydimethylsiloxane

Brand name: Macroplastique

Macroplastique implants are sterile, solid, vulcanized, textured polydimethylsiloxane particles (30% of volume) suspended in a bioexcretable hydrogel carrier.

Much controversy and misconception as well as misunderstanding exist concerning the use of silicones in medical devices. Most of this controversy stems from the Food and Drug Administration (FDA) decision to limit the use of silicone gel-filled breast implants in the United States.[38] However, the empty silicone elastomer breast implants (so called inflatables) are still widely used in the United States, and even the gel-filled mammary implants remain on the major medical markets throughout the world, with very few countries following the FDA's decision.

Silicones are entirely synthetic polymers containing a repeating Si–O backbone and organic groups attached directly to the silicon atom via silicon–carbon bonds. The most common example and the one most commonly used silicone in medical devices is polydimethylsiloxane (PDMS). This is a synthetic polymer with a repeating unit of $(CH_3)_2SiO$.[39] Silicone structural forms and cross-linking allow for the existence of fluids, gels and elastomers.

Fluid silicones are straight chains of PDMS. Silicone gels are lightly cross-linked PDMS, where the cross-linking is achieved with the vinyl and hydrogen groups on separate silicone atoms in the presence of a catalyst. This polymer network is swollen with fluid PDMS to yield a sticky cohesive mass. In the case of silicone gel-filled mammary implants, about 93% of the gel contains fluid PDMS.

Silicone elastomer, on the other hand, is composed of up to 200 PDMS cross-linked radical units. The PDMS elastomer is then usually termed 'solid', polymerized or vulcanized (either at high temperature or room temperature). Usually there is no free fluid polymer.

In 1950, the first implantation of silicone rubber was reported on to replace a urethra.[40] In 1953, silicone was further used for waterproofing skin to prevent maceration.[41] In 1962, the first silastic mammary prosthesis was implanted,[42] and the next year the implantation of silicone sponges and RTV silicone fluid in rats and patients was reported on.[43]

A variety of potential problems have been associated with the use of silicone gel-filled breast implants such as human adjuvant disease,[44–46] scleroderma[47] and systemic lupus erythematosus.[48] However, these few case reports have been associated with silicone gel-filled breast implants. Currently, no reports of any immunological abnormalities in patients that have received inflatable implants or particulate polydimethyl siloxane have been published.[49] The injectable PDMS used in urology (Macroplastique) can only be compared with other fully vulcanized implantable devices such as inflatable mammary implants, but certainly not with silicone gel-filled breast implants (see below).

A recently presented study[50] has hypothesized a possible connection between the use of PDMS micro-implants for the correction of vesico-ureteral reflux and late onset of 'collagen disease'. The hypothesis is based again on observations of patients with gel-filled mammary implants with the presence of migratory silicone present in a finger joint. Three lines of argument are presented to indicate that this study is inconclusive.

First and foremost, the Department of Health (Medical Device Directorate) of the United Kingdom has published, to date, the most comprehensive study summarizing the evidence for an association between the implantation of silicones and connective-tissue disease. The MDD report[49] reviewed all clinical reports of autoimmune disease and 134 relevant publications and concluded that: 'There have been no reported cases of connective tissue disease associated with the use of silicone elastomer devices.'

Secondly, injected or leaking fluid silicone can cause a chronic inflammatory reaction with macrophage vacuolization surrounded by histiocytes and polynuclear giant-cell reaction, diffuse infiltration of lymphocytes and hypertrophic connective tissue.[51] The elastomer micro-implants, by contrast, show a mild foreign-body response (Boros 1A type, non-immunogenic, low turnover).[52,53]

Thirdly, the more cross-linking of PDMS, the higher the biocompatibility. In essence, the length of the polymer chain determines the viscosity. An increase in viscosity is paralleled by the number of units in the chain. As the number of carbon atoms is increased, the material becomes more heat stable and more inert. Fully vulcanized or polymerized PDMS elastomer is therefore completely inert.[51]

The shells of testicular implants, inflatable breast implants, urinary sphincter and penile implant casings, hydrocephalus shunts, finger-joints, intraocular lenses, pacemaker leads and fallopian tube clips are all made of silicone elastomers and there have been no reports of collagen (connective tissue) diseases associated with these implants.[49] In fact, the mere existence of human adjuvants and 'collagen disease' has been severely questioned.[54,55]

The PVP-hydrogel (polyvinylpyrrolidone or povidone), which serves as a carrier medium and lubricant within Macroplastique, has been extensively used in the pharmaceutical, cosmetic and food and beverage industries (Table 1.2).[56] The low-molecular-weight povidone (mean 9800) is biocompatible and is completely excreted through normal glomerular filtration.[56,57] There may be a functional difference with respect to the potential to migrate between the slower excretable povidone within Macroplastique when compared to the vasodilatory properties of the glycerine medium in Polytef.

Biological safety testing on polydimethylsiloxane (Macroplastique)

The particulate PDMS, as well as the hydrogel components of Macroplastique, have undergone considerable biological safety testing on final sterilized products. The following tests were performed to determine the biocompatibility of the vulcanized silicone micro-implants of Macroplastique (data reported in registration file at the Belgian Ministry of Health):

- Haemolysis test. Test to determine the degree of red blood cell lysis and separation of haemoglobin.
- Elution cytotoxicity. Test to determine the lysis of cells, the inhibition of cell growth and other toxic effects.
- Bacterial endotoxins assay. This test estimates the concentration of bacterial endotoxins.

Pharmaceutical uses
- Tablet binder
- Tablet coating
- Ophthalmic preparations
- Topical preparations
- Modification of solubility characteristics of active drug ingredients
- Carrier for transdermal application of drugs
- Germicide in:
  Antimicrobial soaps
  Surgical hand scrubs
  Pre-operative skin cleansers
- Blood plasma expander (during the Second World War)

Foods and beverages
- Blinder for:
  Vitamin concentrate tablets
  Mineral concentrate tablets
  Synthetic sweetener tablets
- Stabilizer for liquid vitamin and mineral concentrates
- Prevents crystallization of liquid synthetic sweetener preparations
- Diluent and dispersant for food colours
- Coating for fresh citrus fruits

Cosmetics and toiletries
Thickener, dispersing agent, lubricant and binder:
  Skin cleansers
  Skin-protection preparations
  Hair tints, dressings, creams
  Stiffener in hair-setting lotions, shampoos, household detergents

Table 1.2. Industrial, pharmaceutical and biological applications of polyvinylpyrrolidone (PVP)

- *Salmonella typhimurium* reverse mutation (Ames) assay. This test evaluates the potential to induce histidine reversion in the genomes of mutant *Salmonella* strains, a bacterial system that evaluates genotoxicity at single-gene level.
- Unscheduled DNA synthesis. The unscheduled deoxyribonucleic acid synthesis assay in primary rat hepatocytes measures the DNA repair synthesis in a section of DNA containing the region of damage possibly induced by a non-autologous material.
- Carcinogenicity assay (*in vitro*). This assay evaluates the carcinogenic potential, which is measured by the ability to cause genetic damage as manifested by induced morphological cell transformation of cell cultures in the absence and presence of an activation system.

- Primary mucosal irritation. This test evaluates the potential to produce a primary irritating effect in conjunction with, or independent of, a corrosive effect.
- Klingman maximization. This biological safety test evaluates the allergic potential or sensitizing capacity.

Test results show that Macroplastique implants are non-haemolytic, have no biological reactivity, were negative of endotoxins and are considered non-mutagenic. In addition, Macroplastique is not considered to be an inducer of unscheduled DNA synthesis in primary hepatocytes, does not induce morphological cell transformation in either activated or non-activated test systems, and is non-irritant and has a grade I sensitization rate which is not considered significant.

Histological findings

To test the suitability of Macroplastique for use as bulking material in urology, in particular paediatric urology, our institute has performed an experimental animal study. Twelve rabbits were injected with 1.0 ml of siloxane micro-implants into the bladder wall and sacrificed at various intervals up to 14 months.

Histological and gross pathological examinations were performed on all major organs including brain, lungs (entire tissue), kidneys, liver, spleen and lymph nodes.

The initial reaction to Macroplastique is characterized by an influx of multi-nucleated cells and fibroblasts (Fig. 1.10). The response then becomes progressively quiescent with the number of multi-nucleated cells decreasing and the fibroblasts maturing into fibrocytes with proto-collagen formation and full maturation at 6–8 weeks (Fig. 1.11). The micro-implants are then fully capsulated in a network of mature collagen fibres (Fig. 1.12).

Examination of the injected sites also showed no abnormal immunogenic response with normal pathological ratings, confirming previously published results.[9,52,53,57,58] A single particle measuring 30 μm in diameter was found within alveoli, with no inflammation or immunogenic abnormalities. A second small particle was identified in the hepatic vein of one of the test animals.

These experimental results are encouraging and confirm earlier results performed on canine models[8,9] that distant migration of these vulcanized silicone micro-implants (Macroplastique) seems to be very limited and may not exist at all.

The biocompatibility of vulcanized PDMS in combination with low-molecular-weight povidone makes this material an excellent choice for endoscopic implantation in urology.

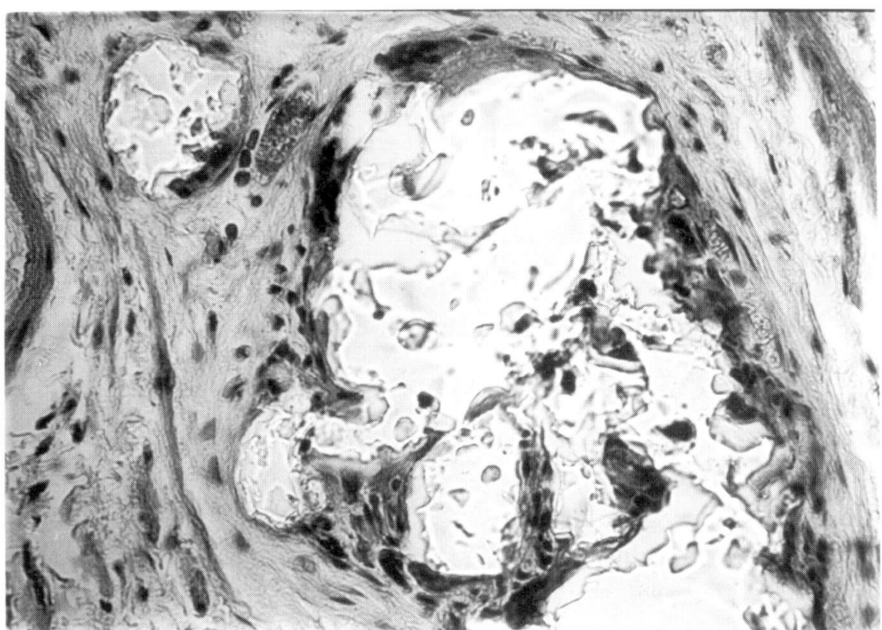

Fig. 1.10. Macroplastique (day 20). Multi-nucleated cells are located in areas directly in contact with the micro-implants. Fibroblasts are maturing and a network of collagen deposits becomes apparent. Few lymphocytes are seen. All Macroplastique particles are completely surrounded by fibrotic collagen deposits.

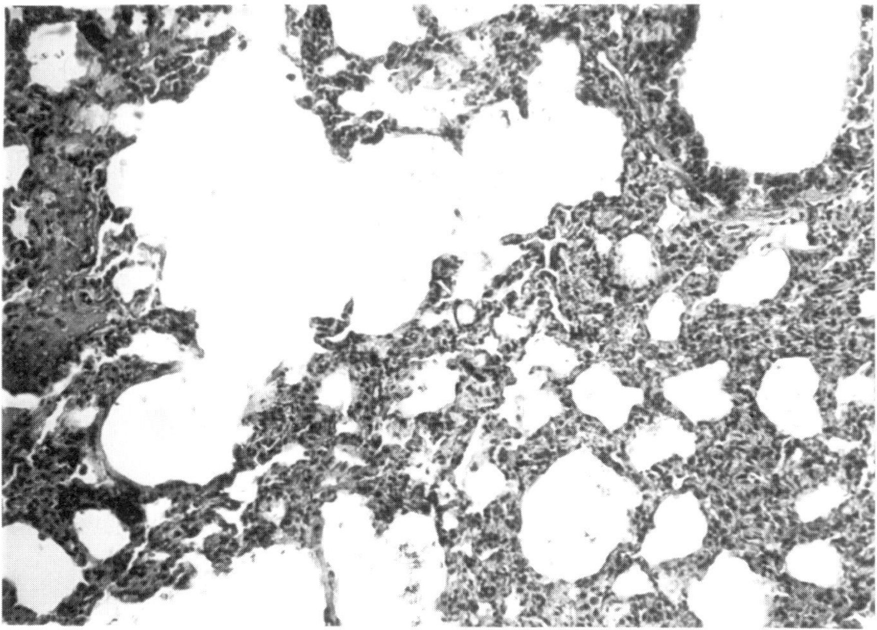

Fig. 1.11. Macroplastique (day 50). More collagen has been laid down by fibroblasts continuing to surround the Macroplastique micro-implants.

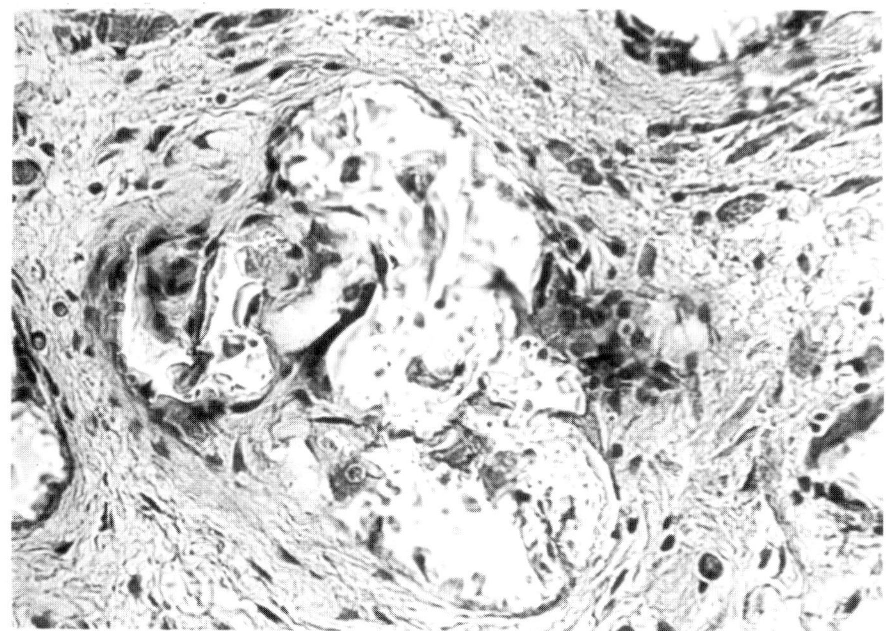

Fig. 1.12. High-power view showing fully encapsulated Macroplastique particles by mature collagen network.

Dextranomer

Brand name: Deflux

Experimental and clinical results[59] report on the use of dextranomer microspheres mixed in a 1% sodium hyalurona (NaHA) solution. Dextranomer microspheres are reported to measure between 40 and 100 μm.

Injections in rat and pig models have shown that the volume of the injection sites decreased after two weeks with an increase in volume after three months.[59] The macroscopical appearance was reported as now showing any mucosal reactions and surrounding tissues were reported as unchanged.

Histopathological analyses demonstrated initially fibroblasts with sparse giant cells surrounding the dextranomers. After three months, there was an ingrowth of fibroblasts, vessels and varying amount of collagen between the dextranomer particles. No typical capsule formation was noticed.[59]

HEMA balloon implants

Brand name: not commercialized

A detachable self-sealing silicone membrane system filled with hydroxyethylmethacrylate (HEMA) has been investigated in pigs for its potential use for the endoscopic correction of reflux.[60] HEMA is a hydrophilic polymer that is compatible with silicone elastomer and which solidifies within 30 min after the addition of ferrous sulphate which was chosen as the filling material. The solidified HEMA can increase the intramural length of the ureters to prevent vesico-ureteral reflux. Until now, no clinical cases have been reported.

Bioglass

Brand name: not commercialized

The safety and biocompatibility of bioglass particles suspended in sodium hyaluronate in rabbits for its use in urology has also been investigated.[61] Until now, however, no clinical cases have been reported.

Ivalon

Brand name: not commercialized

A pilot study investigated the potential use of polyvinyl alcohol foam (Ivalon).[61,62] Particles measuring 150–250 μm were injected into the bladder of New Zealand rabbits. One week after implantation, histological sections showed a foreign body, giant-cell response. At three months, the giant-cell response persisted and particles were surrounded by fibrotic tissue.

Ivalon may induce a considerable fibrotic reaction with granuloma formation similar to Teflon. Tumour growth has also been reported at the implantation site.[63]

Silastic paste

Brand name: not commercialized

An experimental study investigated the effects of an injected silastic paste.[64] The paste is composed of a medical adhesive silicone (type A 7 2947, Dow Corning). The adhesive silastic undergoes a slow polymerization (12–24 hours) when exposed to air and humidity, releasing 6% acetic acid while being solid, but remaining pliable. In the study,[64] 25 rats were injected with the fluid silicone adhesive, with polymerization occurring *in vivo*. Acetic acid is liberated at the mucosal level.

Follow-up studies showed no migration to lymph nodes or other viscera and the granulomatous reactions and fibrotic reaction were milder than in the Teflon control group.

Discussion

The endoscopic treatment of vesico-ureteral reflux is a safe, quick and easily performed, minimally invasive surgery for most cases of reflux. The non-autologous bulking agents herein described each have their own merits from a biocompatible viewpoint, and may differ with respect to their potential for distant migration.

Despite the experimental findings in some studies,[3,10,18,19] no clinical complications or morbidity have been associated to date with the clinical use of the commercially available non-autologous materials Teflon, collagen or Macroplastique. Chapter 2 evaluates the clinical application of these non-autologous injectable materials for the endoscopic correction of reflux.

Acknowledgements

I would like to thank Dr. Mathias Lang (Royal Belgian Institute of Natural Sciences, Brussels) for critical comments.

References

1. Matton G, Anseeuw A, De Keyser F. The history of injectable biomaterials and the biology of collagen. Aesth Plast Surg 1985; 9: 133–40
2. Matouschek E. Die Behandlung des vesikorenalen Refluxes durch transurethrale Einspritzung von Teflonpaste. Urologe 1981; 20: 263–4
3. Malizia AA, Reiman HM, Myers RP et al. Migration and granulomatous reaction after periurethral injection of Polytef (Teflon). JAMA 1984; 251(24): 3277–81
4. Malizia AA, Woodard JR, Rushton HG et al. Intravesical/subureteric injection of Polytef: serial radiology imaging. J Urol 1988; 139: 185A
5. Mittleman RE, Marraccini JV. Pulmonary Teflon granulomas following periurethral Teflon injection for urinary incontinence. [Letter] Arch Pathol Lab Med 1983; 107: 611–12
6. Travis WD, Balogh K, Abraham JL. Silicone granulomas: report of three cases and review of the literature. Human Pathol 1985; 16: 19–27
7. Broutman LJ, Assoc Ltd SEM size distribution analysis of silicone particles in dispensed implants. LJ Broutman & Assoc Ltd Composites and Adhesives Section 1992
8. Henly DR, Barrett DM, Weiland TL et al. Particulate silicone for use in periurethral injections: A study of local tissue effects and a search for migration. Abstracts AUA Meeting Washington DC 1992: 654
9. Smith DP, Kaplan WE. Valuation of polydimethylsiloxane as an alternative in endoscopic treatment of vesicoureteral reflux. Abstract European Urology Congress, Genova, Italy, 1992
10. Vandenbossche M, Delhove O, Dumortier P et al. Endoscopic treatment of reflux: Experimental study and review of Teflon and collagen. Eur Urol 1993; 23: 386–93
11. Politano VA, Small MP, Harper JM et al. Periurethral Teflon injection for urinary incontinence. J Urol 1974; 111: 180
12. O'Donnell B, Puri P. Treatment of vesicoureteral reflux. Br Med J 1984; 289: 7–9
13. Dewan PA. Is injected polytetrafluoroethylene (Polytef) carcinogenic? Br J Urol 1992; 69: 29–33
14. Noe HN, Williams RS, Causay J, Smith DP. Long-term effects of polytetrafluoroethylene injected into the rat bladder submucosa. Urology 1994; 43(6): 852–5
15. Ehrlich RM. Editorial comment. Urology 1994; 43(6): 855–6
16. Claes H, Stroobants D, Van Meerdeek J et al. Pulmonary migration following periurethral polytetrafluoroethylene injection for urinary incontinence. J Urol 1989; 142: 821–2
17. Frey P, Whithaker RH. Prevention of vesicoureteric reflux by endoscopic injection. Br J Urol 1992; 69: 1–6
18. Aaronson IA, Rames RA, Greene WB et al. Endoscopic treatment of reflux: migration of Teflon to the lungs and brain. Eur Urol 1993; 23: 394–9
19. Rames RA, Aaronson IA. Migration of Polytef paste to the lung and brain following intravesical injection for the correction of reflux. Pediatr Surg Int 1991; 6: 239–40
20. Ferro MA, Smith JHF, Smith PJB. Periurethral granuloma: unusual complication of Teflon periurethral injection. Urology 1988; 31(5): 422–3
21. Miyakita H, Puri P. Particles found in lung and brain following subureteral injection of polytetrafluoroethylene paste are not Teflon particles. J Urol 1994; 152: 636–40
22. Lemperle G, Höhler H. Granulome nach Unterspritzung von Gesichtsfalten mit Teflon-Paste. In Höhler H (ed) Plastische und Wiederherstellungschirurgie. Stuttgart, Schattauer. 1975: 335
23. Schulman CC, Pamart D, Hall M et al. Vesicoureteral reflux in children: Endoscopic treatment. Eur Urol 1990; 17: 314–17

24. Marcellin L, Geiss S, Laustriat S et al. Ureteral lesions due to endoscopic treatment of vesicoureteral reflux by injection of Teflon: pathological study. Eur Urol 1990; 17: 325–7

25. Kossovsky N, Millet D, Juma S et al. *In vitro* characterization of the inflammatory properties of poly(tetrafluoroethylene) particulates. J Biomed Mater Res 1992; 25: 1287–1301

26. Hollister DW, Byers PH, Holbrook KA. Genetic disorders of collagen metabolism. In: Harris H, Hirschhorn K (eds) Advances in Human Genetics, 12. New York and London: Plenum Press, 1982

27. Knapp TR, Luck E, Daniels JR. Behaviour of solubilized collagen as a bioimplant. J Surg Res 1977; 23: 96

28. DeLustro F. Overview of the biological response to injectable collagen. 2nd International Congress of Endoscopic Pediatric Urology, October 7–9, 1993. Basel, Switzerland: 37

29. Knapp TR, Kaplan EN, Daniel JR. Injectable collagen for soft tissue augmentation. Plast Reconstr Surg 1977; 60: 398

30. Collagen Corporation: Zyderm collagen implant. Summary of clinical investigation. 1982

31. Stegman SJ, Tromovitch TA. Implantation of collagen for depressed scars. J Dermatol Surg Oncol 1980; 6: 450

32. Schumrick KA, Kridel RWH. Comparison of injectable silicone versus collagen for soft tissue augmentation. J Dermatol Surg Oncol 1988; 14(1): 66–72

33. Kaplan EN, Falces E, Tolleth H. Clinical utilization of injectable collagen. Ann Plast Surg 1983; 10: 437–51

34. Lemperle G, Ott H, Charrier U et al. PMMA microspheres for intradermal implantation: Part I. Animal Research. Ann Plast Surg 1991; 26(1): 57–63

35. Frey P. A new injectable collagen for the endoscopic treatment of vesicoureteric reflux and incontinence. An experimental study in the mini-pig. 2nd International Congress of Endoscopic Pediatric Urology, October 7–9, 1993. Basel, Switzerland: 38

36. Lipsky H. Endoscopic treatment of vesicoureteric reflux with bovine collagen. Eur Urol 1990; 18: 52–5

37. Leonard MP, Canning DA, Epstein JI et al. Local tissue reaction to the subureteral injection of glutaraldehyde cross-linked bovine collagen in humans. J Urol 1990; 143: 1209–12

38. Kessler DA. The basis of the FDA's decision on breast implants. New Engl J Med 1992; 326(25): 1713–15

39. LeVier RR. What is silicone? Plast Reconstr Surg 1993; 92(1): 163–7

40. De Nicola RR. Permanent artificial (silicone) urethra. J Urol 1950; 63: 168

41. Brown JB, Fryer MP, Randall P, Lu M. Silicones in plastic surgery. Plast Reconstr Surg 1973; 47: 343

42. Gerow FJ, Spira M, Hardy SB, Law S. Silicone immersion treatment of the severely burned patient. In: Transactions of the Third International Congress of Plastic Surgery. Amsterdam: Excerpta Medica Foundation. 1963: 146

43. Speirs AC, Blocksma R. New implantable silicone rubbers. Plast Reconstr Surg 1963; 31: 166

44. Byron MA, Venning V, Mowat AG. Case report: Post-mammoplasty human adjuvant disease. Br J Rheumatol 1984; 23: 227–9

45. Weisman MH, Vecchione TR, Albert D et al. Connective tissue disease following breast augmentation: a preliminary test of the human adjuvant disease hypothesis. Plast Reconstr Surg 1988; 4: 626–30

46. Brozena SJ, Fenske NA, Cruse CW et al. Observations: human adjuvant disease following augmentation mammoplasty. Arch Dermatol 1988; 124: 1383–6

47. Sahn EE, Garen PD, Silver RM, Maize JC. Observations: Scleroderma following augmentation mammoplasty. Arch Dermatol 1990; 126: 1198–1222

48. Jacobs JC, Imundo LF. [Letter to the editor] Lancet 1994: 354–5

49. Tinkler JJB, Campbell HJ, Senior JM, Ludgate SM. Evidence for an association between the implantation of silicones and connective tissue disease. Medical Device Directorate (UK Department of Health) Report 1993; MDD/92/42: 1–65

50. Aaronson IA, Silver RM, Greene WB. Children with reflux treated by Macroplastique may be at risk for late onset collagen disease. Abstract ESPU 5th Annual Meeting 1994; 20: 1–2

51. Habal MB. The biological basis for the clinical applications of the silicones. Arch Surg 1984; 119: 843–8

52. Beisang AA, Ersek RA. Mammalian response to subdermal implantation of textured microimplants. Aesth Plast Surg 1992; 16: 83–90

53. Allen O. Response to subdermal implantation of textured microimplants in humans. Aesth Plast Surg 1992; 16: 227–30

54. Brody GS, Conway DP, Deapen DM et al. Consensus statement on the relationship of breast implants to connective-tissue disorders. Plast Reconstr Surg 1992; 90(6): 1102–4

55. Sanchez-Guerrero J, Liang MH. Silicone breast implants and connective tissue diseases. No association has been convincingly established. Br Med J 1994; 309: 822–3

56. Robinson BV, Sullivan FM, Borzelleca JF, Schwartz SL. PVP: A critical review of the kinetics and toxicology of polyvinylpyrrolidone (Povidone). Chelsea, MI: Lewis Publishers, Inc, 1990.

57. Laing JHE, Sanders R. The Misti Gold bio-oncotic gel filled breast prosthesis: an acceptable alternative to silicone? Br J Plast Surg 1993; 44: 240–2

58. Dewan PA, Byard RW. Histological response to injected Polytef and Bioplastique in a rat model. Br J Urology 1994; 73: 370–6

59. Stenberg A, Läckgren G. Endoscopic treatment of vesicoureteral reflux with subureteric injection of a new tissue-augmenting biodegradable substance. Preliminary results. 2nd International Congress of Endoscopic Pediatric Urology. October 7–9, 1993. Basel, Switzerland: 16.

60. Atala A, Peters CA, Retik AB, Mandell J. Endoscopic treatment of vesicoureteral reflux with a self-detachable balloon system. J Urol 1992; 148: 724–7

61. Walker RD, Wilson J, Clark AE. Injectable bioglass as a potential substitute for injectable polytetrafluoroethylene. J Urol 1992; 148: 645–7

62. Merguerian PA, McLorie GA, Khoury AE et al. Submucosal injection of polyvinyl alcohol foam in rabbit bladder. J Urol 1990; 144: 531–3

63. Canning DA. New implants for endoscopic correction of vesicoureteral reflux in the nineties and beyond. Dialogues Pediatr Urol 1991; 14(2): 6–8

64. Valla JS, Hofman P, Pallanca G et al. Etude expérimentale sur les injections vésicales sous-muqueuses chez le rat. Téflon contre silicone. J Urologie 1989; 95(8): 471–5

Non-autologous injected materials for the endoscopic treatment of vesico-ureteral reflux

2

C. C. Schulman

Introduction

Persistent vesico-ureteral reflux can result in progressive renal damage and ultimately lead to renal failure. The main treatment choices are either administration of prophylactic antibiotics, open surgery or endoscopic submucosal implantations.

The principle of endoscopic correction of vesico-ureteral reflux is to create a solid support behind the intravesical ureter by endoscopic injection of materials, thereby elongating the intramural length of the ureter. The additional trajectory and the extrinsic pressure is, in most cases, sufficient to protect the ureterovesical (UV) junction from reflux.

The subureteric injection methodology for reflux was first reported in 1981[1] and applied to both the bladder neck and ureters.[2] The endoscopic treatment was further popularized in the mid-to-late 1980s and became known as the subureteric Teflon injection (STING) procedure.[3,4] The injection technique is simple and can be performed as a day-case procedure, but does require a certain, be it short, learning curve. Scope time itself varies from 5 to 15 min depending on the proficiency of the surgeon and the positioning of ureteral orifices, degree of reflux and uni- or bilateral indications.

The use of non-autologous injectable substances, however, for the treatment of vesico-ureteral reflux and which material is most appropriate is still debated quite vigorously. The disadvantages of non-autologous materials mentioned have included particle migration with subsequent volume loss at the injection site, granuloma formation and possible latent carcinogenic effects.

Success in endoscopic therapy may depend more upon the positioning of the implants and the amount used, as well as patient selection, than on the choice of materials. Experience has shown that the appropriate position is inside the periureteral sheath of the intramural ureter just proximal to the ureteral orifices. Failures can be attributed to injections into the subserosal layers of the bladder wall, the detrusor musculature, ureteral lumen or extravesically as well as a shifting of the injected materials after implantation or simply too far from the ureteral orifice and too little material injected.

Equipment and components

A variety of permutations of equipment (scopes, guns, needles, lubricants) can be used for the injection therapy. Needles are either rigid or flexible depending on the type of endoscopes used.

Classical straight-viewing cystoscopes require flexible needles. The most commonly used injection needles are 5 Fr flexible needles (35-cm long) with a 7-mm rigid needle of either a 20 gauge (Uroplasty Inc.) used for Macroplastique or a 23 or 25 gauge (Cook Urological, Bard) used for Teflon and collagen. The larger bore needle tip is required for Macroplastique because of the larger average particle size (180 µm). The smallest straight-viewing scope that can be used with these needles is a 13.5 Fr endoscope. Preferably however, a 15 Fr should be considered as minimum size. The advantage of using a flexible needle is that it can be manipulated with the deflector (Albaran or bridge). A disadvantage is that one person has to manipulate the scope and direct the needle from the distal end of the scope while the other person has to 'follow' the endoscope to prevent kinking of the needle at the distal end of the cystoscope and to aid in injecting.

On the other hand, an 'angled' scope with a straight-working channel and offset lens (either fixed or movable) requires a rigid needle. The most commonly used rigid needles are stainless steel, again with either a 20, 23 or 25 gauge 7-mm tip, depending on the material to be injected. The advantage of this set-up is that a single surgeon can direct the scope with one hand and direct the needle and attached injection instrument with the other. An additional advantage is that smaller scopes (as small as 9.5 Fr) can be used.

Injectors range from a simple syringe (collagen) to a ratchet gun (Macroplastique and Teflon) to a hand-held battery-powered high-pressure injector (Teflon). The existing Teflon injection system in most medical units consists of a hand-held Storz gun syringe and needle (see above). The injection syringe is small (1 ml), very difficult to fill, and requires periodic refilling. The Macroplastique injection system consists of a prefilled sterile syringe (3 ml syringe filled to 1.8 ml with 1.3 ml usable material), a flexible or rigid needle and an injector gun. The injector gun is a hand-held ratchet type with piston, advanced by trigger, and syringe holder. The piston is advanced by pulling the trigger.

Endoscopic technique

Under direct vision through the cystoscope, the needle tip is introduced up to 7-mm distal to the affected ureteral orifice into the periureteral space at the 6 o'clock position. The needle tip is advanced about 4–5 mm into the lamina propria of the submucosal portion of the ureter and the injection is started slowly. As the injection proceeds, care should be taken to both

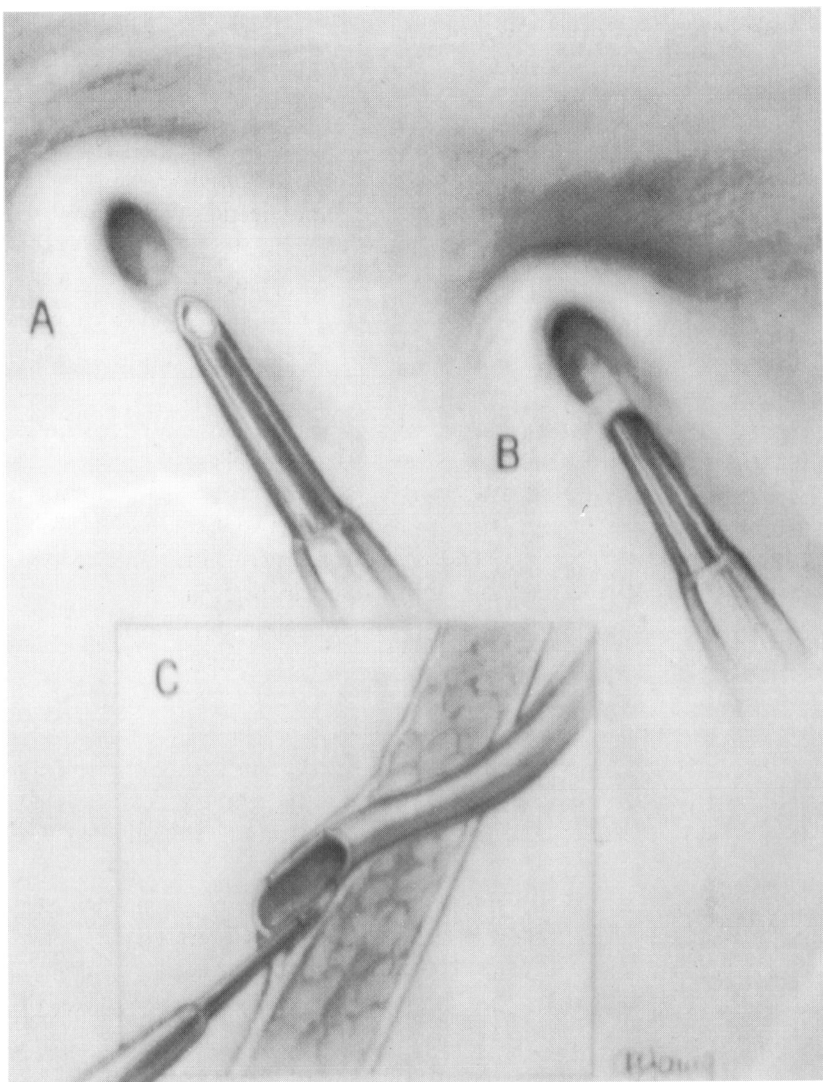

Fig. 2.1. Subureteric needle placement. (A) Needle is positioned at the 6 o'clock position. (B) Needle insertion into the subureteric space. (C) Cut-away view to indicate the placement of the needle prior to injection. (From Kaplan, 1987[36].)

check visually for mucosal elevation and manually monitor pressure on the injector gun or syringe. If the resistance pressure drops without mucosal elevation, then the needle positioning is inaccurate. Slow continual pressure should elevate the mucosa so that the orifice lies on the summit of a small mound and assumes an inverted crescent appearance at the end of the procedure (Fig. 2.1). During injection (Fig. 2.2), the needle tip may be withdrawn slightly to achieve better mucosal elevation if necessary. The

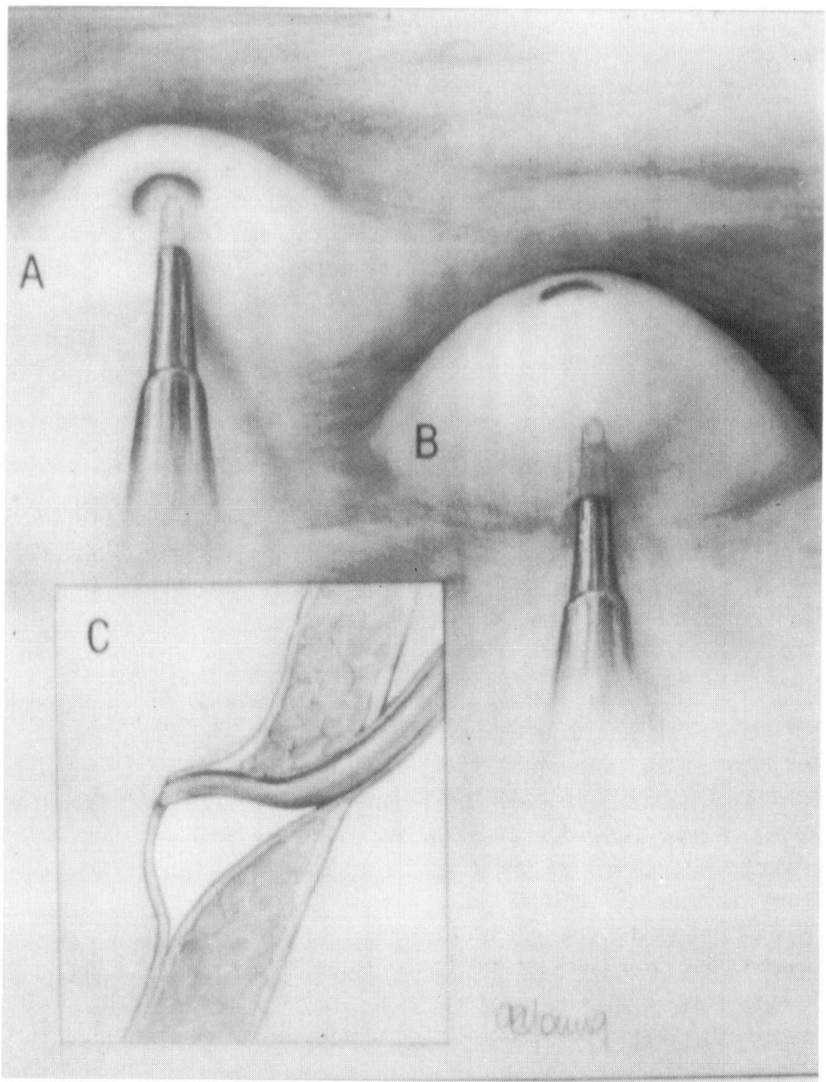

Fig. 2.2. Injection of material. (A) Initial injection is made to create a small hillock. Note that the injection of substance should always be associated with mucosal elevation. (B) Final result with inverted crescent-shaped ureteral orifice at summit of mound. (C) Cut-away view of final placement of injected material. (From Kaplan, 1987[36].)

needle tip should be kept in place for some time (5 s for Macroplastique and collagen; 30–60 s for Teflon) to avoid extrusion of implanted material.

If the mound appears in an incorrect place, e.g. off to the side of the ureter or proximal to it, the needle should be repositioned so that the end result is that the orifice lies at the summit of the mound of injected material. Either the initial mucosal entrance site or a new one can be used.

The amount of material to be injected varies due to bulging properties of material used, the positioning of the needle, the grade of reflux (i.e. condition of the ureteral orifice) and the expansibility of the mucosa.

Some discussion as to the appropriate follow-up exists. The Dublin group[3,5–11] has the longest experience with this technique and recommends the prescription of the preoperative antibiotic for 6–12 weeks after the procedure. Micturating cystourethrography (MCU) and ultrasonography is recommended three months after discharge. Follow-up MCUs are at one year and again at three years after the endoscopic correction of reflux.[12]

Results: materials and indications

Materials

Three types of materials are predominantly used in the endoscopic treatment of vesico-ureteral reflux: polytetrafluoroethylene (Polytef); collagen; and Macroplastique. Table 2.1 provides a comparative overview of various aspects of these three different materials.

Teflon	Collagen	Macroplastique
Migration	Immunological reactions	Limited migration
Granuloma	Non-permanent	Inert
Good results	Moderate results	Good results

Table 2.1. Materials used in the endoscopic treatment of vesico-ureteral reflux. There is no ideal material and there have been no clinical complications to date

Polytetrafluoroethylene/Teflon/Polytef
Procedure: STING (subureteric Teflon injection)

Polytef consists of 33% polytetrafluoroethylene, 33% glycerine and 33% polysorbate. The polytetrafluoroethylene particles have an irregular surface and range from 4 to 100 μm in diameter, with more than 90% of the particles in the Teflon paste ranging from 4 to 40 μm in diameter.[13]

Glycerine is used as lubricant. It is also available as glyceryl trinitrate, a powerful vasodilator with a short action (20–30 min) and as glycerol suppositories, which maintain fluid levels in the large bowel by osmosis and vasodilation. The glycerine lubricant, because of its vasodilatory properties, is absorbed very quickly probably taking the smaller particles of Teflon as well. The remaining Teflon particles are usually encapsulated in their entirety with no collagen deposits between the individual particles.

Collagen/Gax-Collagen/Atelocollagen
Procedure: SCIN (subureteric collagen injection).

Injectable collagen is composed of purified bovine dermal collagen

(3.5% by volume) that is cross-linked with glutaraldehyde and dispersed in phosphate-buffered physiological saline.

PDMS (polydimethylsiloxane)
Procedure: SUMMIT (subureteric microparticulate Macroplastique injection therapy).

Macroplastique consists of solid polydimethylsiloxane particles (30% of volume) in a bio-excretable hydrogel carrier (non-iodine Povidone).

Indications
Each individual surgeon has his or her own criteria in selecting patients for endoscopic treatment of reflux. Table 2.2 gives a broad range of patient-selection criteria. Success rates themselves depend on the indications treated. As discussed below, variable successes are achieved in patient populations with different grades of reflux (I to II versus IV and V); duplicated systems versus non-duplicated primary refluxing systems, neurogenic versus normal compliant bladders and the location of the ureteral orifices with the amount of tissue support. Periureteral diverticula are extremely difficult to correct because of lack of adequate detrusor muscle support.

Tables 2.3, 2.4 and 2.5 provide recent selected published results of endoscopic correction of reflux for indications of primary and secondary treatment of reflux in children using three different materials. However, it seems that in the pre-1990 studies, success rates were slightly lower.

A 1986 study of the Dublin group[6] indicated a 75% success rate after one injection. In a 1987 study[27] 99 of 153 ureters (65%) had absence of reflux on postmicturation voiding cystourethrography after endoscopic correction with Teflon.

The most recent studies indicate that for primary and secondary treatment of reflux by endoscopic means a success rate of over 90% is achievable when using Macroplastique or Teflon, whereas the success rate with collagen is somewhat lower (Table 2.3). About 65% of refluxing ureters are cured after the first injection.[17,20] These results perhaps reflect the rapid absorption of the physiological saline carrier. As with Teflon, a

---

- All grades of reflux
- Poor prophylactic compliance
- Patients with antibiotic resistance
- Failed ureteral reimplantation
- Thick-walled neurogenic bladder
- Persistent reflux after augmentation and/or reconstruction procedures
- Refluxing renal transplant recipients with poor tissue healing

---

Table 2.2. Endoscopic correction of vesico-ureteral reflux. Patient selection

Reference	Year	After 1st injection	After 2nd injection	No. of injections unknown
O'Donnel and Puri [3]	1984	77%	94%	
Schulman [4]	1987	88%	97%	
Dodat [26]	1990	85%	89%	
Sauvage [25]	1990			92%
Farkas [23]	1990	94%	98%	
Geiss [21]	1990			82%
Borowka [19]	1991			91%
Schulman [18]	1992	87%	93%	
Nakajima [16]	1993	63%	93%	

Table 2.3. Endoscopic correction of primary and secondary reflux. Teflon

Reference	Year	After 1st injection	After 2nd injection	No. of injections unknown
Lipsky [22]	1990			86%
Leonard [20]	1991			65%
Frey [17]	1992	68%	90%	

Table 2.4. Endoscopic correction of primary and secondary reflux. Collagen (1990–1994)

Reference	Year	After 1st injection	After 2nd injection	No. of injections unknown
Buckley [15]	1993			91% downgraded: 4%
Dodat [14]	1994	91%	97%	

Table 2.5. Endoscopic correction of primary and secondary reflux. Macroplastique

second injection may increase the cure rate, which then again may be reduced over time.[20,28] Failure of a SCIN may not only be due to the reabsorption of the carrier medium and degradation of the collagen by collagenase but possibly also due to the tendency of the bolus to become displaced from the ureteral orifices to the bladder neck by the muscular contractions of the trigone during voiding.[29]

Reflux into duplex ureters was corrected in 82% of patients after first injection and 93% after repeated injections[23] and 58% and 74%, respectively, in another study[24] (Table 2.6). An earlier study involved patients with ureteral duplication; this was more difficult to correct and treat, with only 50% success.[35] Reported resolution[36] of reflux in patients with neurogenic bladder dysfunction of 84% after one injection of Teflon, improving to 87% after a second injection, has been substantiated by two more recent studies (Table 2.6).

A recent multi-centre study[12] reports on the results from 18 centres in Europe with a total of 6216 refluxing uterers using Teflon. Success rate (i.e.

Reference	Year	Material	After 1st injection	After 2nd injection
Farkas [23]	1990	Teflon	82%	93%
Schulman [4]	1990	Teflon	58%	74%
Geiss [21]	1990	Teflon		70%*
Neurogenic bladder dysfunction				
Hashimoto [30]	1994	Teflon	100% at first injection (16% downgraded over time: 25 months)	
Kaminetsky [31]	1991	Teflon	70% (3-year postoperative follow-up)	
Geiss [21]	1990	Teflon	70%	

Table 2.6. Endoscopic correction of reflux. Specific conditions. Duplex ureters
*Number of injections unknown

• Number of centres	18
• Number of ureters	6216
• Follow-up	90% followed for 2 years
• Mean age	5.2 years
• Grades	I to V
• Cured	76% after 1st injection → 85% after 2nd injection
• Downgraded	10%
• Failure	4%
• Obstruction	0.3% (reimplanted without difficulty)

Table 2.7. Endoscopic correction of reflux. Teflon. (After Puri, 1995, in press)

no reflux) following the first injection was 76.3% and increased to 84.9% after a second treatment. The long-term success is less certain, because among the centres in which follow-up cystograms (one or more years after implantation) have been carried out, a relapse rate of between 9 and 15% has been noted[9,37,38]. This suggests that an average permanent cure rate with Teflon for all the above-mentioned indications may lie around 75% (Table 2.7).

Complications: surgical versus endoscopic

Surgical

Complications after ureteral reimplantation result from either preoperative planning errors or errors in intraoperative technique.[39] Excessive tissue handling during ureteral mobilization may contribute to postoperative oedema or devascularization of the ureter. Technical errors during the surgical intervention can include ureteral perforation, ureteral transection or avulsion during mobilization, ureteral obstruction secondary to the creation of a too tight detrusor hiatus, passing the ureter through a peritoneal fold or intraperitoneal structure, and placement of the neohiatus too cranially and laterally on the posterior surface of the bladder.

Early perioperative complications include bleeding, sepsis, catheter obstruction or dislodgement, ureteral obstruction, annuria and prolonged ileus.[39] The incidence of uretero-vesical obstruction requiring reoperation is estimated at between 1.2 and 4%. The cause of obstruction after surgical reimplantation is usually due to mechanical factors, ischaemia or an unrecognized 'neuropathic bladder'. The incidence of persistent vesico-ureteral reflux requiring reoperation ranges between 1 and 3%. The failure here is due primarily to either a submucosal tunnel that is too short or an unrecognized neuropathic bladder.[39]

In a well-documented study,[40] 20% of surgically reimplanted patients demonstrated failure between 4 and 10 years after initial ureteral re-implantation. Because obstruction is likely to be a late serious complication, it is imperative to follow patients carefully after ureteral reimplantation. Periodic ultrasonic examinations of the urinary tract are advised.

The majority of failed ureteral reimplantations either secondary to uretero-vesical junction obstruction or secondary to reflux can be salvaged by using well-described techniques. Occasionally, a ureter can become atonic, scarred and shortened after multiple attempts at reimplantation.[39] Selected patients may require an augmentation cystoplasty to alter bladder dynamics or for reimplantation of the refluxing ureter into the bowel segment.

Laparoscopic vesico-ureteroplasty

In a recent study, operating times of 2 hours 15 minutes and 3 hours 15 minutes were recorded for a laparoscopic vesico-ureteroplasty operation on two patients. This procedure certainly has the major advantages over the surgical technique in being a minimally invasive therapy and is perhaps a technique to be looked towards in the near future. No complications were noted here.

Endoscopic treatment

Procedure-related complications of endoscopic correction of reflux are rare. Transient side effects of dysuria, frequency and haematuria are sometimes noted in the first day or two after endoscopic implantation. A recent European survey involving 6216 ureters in 4166 patients revealed vesico-ureteric obstruction in only 20 ureters (0.0003%).[12] There have been no major reports or evidence of upper-tract (kidney) obstruction or serious clinical complications using this technique. In addition, the short hospitalization time severely reduces the peri- and postoperative pain.

For failures of an initial endoscopic correction of reflux (for causes, see above), a second implantation technique is recommended. Failures of a secondary treatment can still be treated by surgical reimplantation without any complications. In fact, the only significant complication with this procedure remains the failure to abolish reflux at the initial injection.

Migration

Some physicians have been concerned by the use of non-autologous materials, in particular polytetrafluoroethylene, because distant migration after periurethral, periureteral and intravenous injection has been reported in animal studies.[13,42,43] A recent detailed experimental study[44] in two different animal models investigated whether particles of polytetrafluoroethylene migrated to the lungs and brain following subureteral, intravenous or intra-arterial injection. Animals with Teflon particles injected into the submucosal plane showed no signs of migration. On the other hand, animals with intravenous injection of Teflon particles showed Teflon to be present in the lungs and not the brain, and animals with Teflon particles injected directly into the carotid artery showed the presence of polytetrafluoroethylene in the brain on histological examination. Table 2.6 lists selected references indicating migration of Teflon particles in humans.

Additional experimental studies[48,49] have shown very limited migration of large particulated Macroplastique implants. The few particles that migrated were suggested to be the result of the injection technique (i.e. implanted extravesically), which in laboratory animals is much more difficult than in humans.

Summary and conclusions

Endoscopic correction of vescico-ureteral reflux is an appealing technique for patients with persistent vesico-ureteral reflux as a primary choice. It is also useful in patients with poor prophylactic compliance, in patients after failed ureteral reimplantation, in selected patients with neuropathic bladder dysfunction in whom open surgical techniques are less likely to produce a successful result, or in patients with persistent reflux after complicated augmentation or reconstruction procedures. Endoscopic treatment of vesico-ureteral reflux is also particularly appealing in children with high-grade reflux and neuropathic vesical dysfunction. Furthermore, endoscopic treatment does not complicate or preclude open surgery at a later date.

Long-term antibiotic prophylaxis is difficult to monitor and there are often problems with compliance. The submucosal injection of Teflon has good early and long-term results but because of some safety concerns about Teflon (migration and progressive fibrosis) its use has been diminished. Injectable collagen has been quite promising but early recurrence has been reported due to autodigestion of the collagen. Macroplastique, on the other hand, has good bulking properties, requiring less material with limited or non-existent migration of the comparatively large inert microparticles.

Although the results of endoscopic correction of reflux are slightly inferior to those of open surgery, endoscopic correction of vesico-ureteral reflux has been shown to be much safer than surgical treatment in terms of possible complications. In fact, the only significant complication with the endoscopic procedure remains the failure to abolish reflux at the initial injection. In addition, there is minimal hospitalization required and future surgery is not precluded.

Acknowledgement

Dr. Mathias Lang (Royal Belgian Institute of Natural Sciences, Department of Recent Vertebrates) is thanked for critical comments.

References

1. Matouschek E. Die Behandlung des vesikorenalen Refluxes durch transurethrale Einspritzung von Teflonpaste. Urologe 1981; 20: 263–4
2. Politano VA. Periurethral polytetrafluoroethylene injection for urinary incontinence. J Urol 1982; 127: 439–42
3. O'Donnell B, Puri P. Treatment of vesicoureteral reflux. Br Med J 1984; 289: 7–9
4. Schulman CC, Simon J, Pamart D, Avni FE. Endoscopic treatment of vesicoureteral reflux in children. J Urol 1987; 138: 950
5. O'Donnell B, Puri P. Endoscopic correction of primary vesicoureteric reflux. Results in 94 ureters. Br Med J 1986; 293: 1404–6
6. O'Donnell B, Puri P. Endoscopic correction of primary vesicoureteric reflux. Br J Urol 1986; 58: 601
7. Puri P, Guiney EJ. Endoscopic correction of vesicoureteric reflux secondary to neuropathic bladder. Br J Urol 1986; 58: 504–6
8. Puri P, O'Donnell B. Endoscopic correction of primary vesicoureteric reflux of grades IV and V. J Ped Surg 1987; 22: 1087–91
9. Puri P. Endoscopic correction of primary vesicoureteric reflux by STING – follow-up study in 123 patients. Pediatr Surg Int 1991; 6: 269–72
10. Puri P. Endoscopic correction of primary vesicoureteric reflux by subureteric injection of polytetrafluoroethylene. Lancet 1990; 335: 1320–2
11. Miyakita H, Ninan GK, Puri P. Endoscopic correction of vesicoureteric reflux in duplex systems. Eur Urol 1993; 24: 111–15
12. Ninan GK, Puri P. Subureteric Teflon injection (STING): Results of a European survey. Presented at the Annual Meeting of the British Association of Urological Surgeons, Harrogate, June 1993
13. Malizia AA, Reiman HM, Myers RP et al. Migration and granulomatous reaction after periurethral injection of Polytef (Teflon). JAMA 1984; 251(24): 3277–81
14. Dodat H. Traitement endoscopique du reflux vésicorénal chez l'enfant. Arch Pédiatr 1994; 1: 93–100
15. Buckley JF, Azmy AA, Fyfe AB et al. Endoscopic correction of vesico-ureteric reflux with injectable silicone microparticles. J Urol 1993; 149: 259
16. Nakajima H, Ando T, Ujiie T et al. Endoscopic correction of vesicoureteral reflux by Teflon. Hinyokika-Kiyo 1993; 39(7): 599–603
17. Frey P, Berger D, Jenny P, Herzog B. Subureteral collagen injection for the endoscopic treatment of vesicoureteral reflux in children. Follow-up study of 97 treated ureters and histological analysis of collagen implants. J Urol 1992; 148: 718–23
18. Schulman CC, Sassine AM. Endoscopic treatment of vesicoureteral reflux. Eur J Pediatr Surg 1992; 2(1): 32–4
19. Borowka A, Hanecki R, Kuzaka B et al. Early results of endoscopic treatment of vesico-ureteral reflux in children. Urologe-A 1991; 30(4): 264–6
20. Leonard MP, Canning DA, Peters CA et al. Endoscopic injection of glutaraldehyde cross-

linked bovine dermal collagen for correction of vesicoureteral reflux. J Urol 1991; 145(1): 115–19

21. Geiss S, Alessandrini P, Allouch G et al. Multicenter survey of endoscopic treatment of vesicoureteral reflux in children. Eur Urol 1990; 17(4): 328–9

22. Lipsky H. Endoscopic treatment of vesicoureteric reflux with bovine collagen. Eur Urol 1990; 18(1): 52–5

23. Farkas A, Moriel EZ, Lupa S. Endoscopic correction of vesicoureteral reflux: our experience with 115 ureters. J Urol 1990; 144: 534–6

24. Schulman CC, Pamart D, Hall M et al. Vesicoureteral reflux in children: endoscopic treatment. Eur Urol 1990; 17(4): 314–17

25. Sauvage P, Geiss S, Saussine C et al. Analysis and perspectives of endoscopic treatment of vesicoureteral reflux in children with a 20-month follow-up. Eur Urol 1990; 17(4): 310–13

26. Dodat H, Takvorian P. Treatment of vesicoureteral reflux in children by endoscopic injection of Teflon: Review of 2 years of experience. Eur Urol 1990; 17(4): 304–6

27. Sweeny LE, Thomas PS. Evaluation of sub-ureteric Teflon injection as an antireflux procedure. Ann Radiol (Paris) 1987; 30: 478

28. Capozza N, Caione P, De Gennaro M, Patricolo M. Endoscopic treatment of vesico-ureteral reflux (VUR) and urinary incontinence: Technical problems in the pediatric patient. ESPU 5th Annual Meeting, Göteborg. 1994; Abstract 35

29. Reunanen MS. Correction of vesicorenal reflux in children by collagen injection; a 5 year follow-up with correlation to ureteral function, ureteral location and duplication. ESPU 5th Annual Meeting. Göteborg. 1994; Abstract 85

30. Hashimoto K, Kishima Y, Onishi N et al. Transurethral Teflon paste injection for vesicoureteral reflux in neurogenic bladder dysfunction. Nippon-Hinyokika-Gakkai-Zasshi 1993; 84(12): 2118–23

31. Kaminetsky JC, Hanna MK. Endoscopic treatment of vesicoureteral reflux in children with neurogenic bladders. Urology 1991; 37(3): 244–7

32. Gonzalez-Martin M, Sousa-Escandon A, Busto-Castonon L et al. Endoscopic treatment of vesicoureteral reflux following transurethral resection of a vesical carcinoma by Teflon injection. Eur Urol 1991; 19(4): 291–4

33. Kohri K, Imanishi M, Kunikata S et al. Investigation on unsuccessful endoscopic operation for cases with vesicoureteral reflux. Nippon-Hinyokika-Gakkai-Zasshi 1992; 83(12): 1964–9

34. Sironvalle MS, Gelet A, Martin X et al. Endoscopic treatment of vesicoureteral reflux prior to renal transplantation. Transpl Inr 1992; 5(4): 231–3

35. Quinlan D, O'Donnell B. Unilateral ureteric reimplantation for primary vesicoureteric reflux in children. Br J Urol 1985; 57: 406

36. Kaplan WE, Dalton DP, Firlit CF. The endoscopic correction of reflux by polytetrafluoroethylene injection. J Urol 1987; 138: 953–5

37. Sauvage P, Geiss S, Dhaoui R et al. Analysis and technical refinements of endoscopic treatment of vesicoureteral reflux in children with a 40 month follow-up. Pediatr Surg Int 1991; 6: 277–80

38. Dodat H, Takvorian P, Sabatier E et al. Treatment of vesicoureteral reflux in children by endoscopic injection of Teflon. Review of $3\frac{1}{2}$ years experience. Pediatr Surg Int 1991; 6: 273–6

39. Kramer SE. Vesicoureteral reflux. In: Kelalis PP, King LR, Belman AB (eds) Clinical Pediatric Urology. London: W.B. Saunders, 1992; 441–99

40. Mesrobian H-Gj, Kramer SA, Kelalis PP. Reoperative ureteroneocystostomy: review of 69 patients. J Urol 1985; 133: 388

41. Ehrlich RM, Gershman A, Fuchs G. Laparoscopic vesicoureteroplasty in children: initial case reports. Urology 1994; 43(2): 255–61

42. Rames RA, Aaronson IA. Migration of Polytef paste to the lung and brain following intravesical injection for the correction of reflux. Pediatr Surg Int 1991; 6: 239–40

43. Aaronson IA, Rames RA, Greene WB et al. Endoscopic treatment of reflux: migration of Teflon to the lungs and brain. Eur Urol 1993; 23: 394–9

44. Miyakita H, Puri P. Particles found in lung and brain following subureteral injection of polytetrafluoroethylene paste are not Teflon particles. J Urol 1994; 152: 636–40

45. Mittleman RE, Marraccini JV. Pulmonary Teflon granulomas following periurethral Teflon injection for urinary incontinence [Letter]. Arch Pathol Lab Med 1983; 107: 611–12

46. Kaufman M, Lockhart JL, Silverstein MJ, Politano VE. Transurethral polytetrafluoroethylene injection for postprostatectomy incontinence. J Urol 1084; 132: 463–4
47. Claes H, Stroobants D, Van Meerdeek J et al. Pulmonary migration following periurethral polytetrafluorethylene injection for urinary incontinence. J Urol 1989; 142: 821–2
48. Henly DR, Barrett DM, Weiland TL et al. Particulate silicone for use in periurethral injections: A study of local tissue effects and a search for migration. Abstracts AUA Meeting Washington DC 1992: 654
49. Smith DP, Kaplan WE, Oyasu R. Evaluation of polydimethylsiloxane as an alternative in the endoscopic treatment of vesicoureteral reflux. J Urol 1994; 152: 1221–4

Surgical procedures, indications and results of injected materials for treating urinary incontinence (male and female)

3

G. Williams

Introduction

The International Continence Society has defined urinary incontinence as the involuntary loss of urine that is objectively demonstrated and a social hygienic problem.[1] Based on American figures, the annual cost of treating incontinence is estimated at billions of dollars per annum.[2] In 1992, the United States agency for health care, policy and research published its guidelines for urinary incontinence. Their main points were that urinary incontinence is a common and often neglected condition, that treatment should be offered in stepwise fashion beginning with the least invasive therapy and that the cause of incontinence should be documented objectively before surgical treatment is undertaken.

Urinary incontinence has been the subject of some unhelpful classifications and irrelevant urodynamic studies. Excluding fistulas, the only two conditions which cause incontinence are uncontrolled bladder contractility and urethral sphincter dysfunction.

Physiology of continence

The urethra functions, not only as a conduit for urine (and seminal fluid in men), but also a sphincter resisting the forces of intravesical and intra-abdominal pressure to maintain continence. Continence is achieved because the maximal urethral pressure is greater than the intravesical pressure when the bladder fills and because rises in intra-abdominal pressure are transmitted equally to the vesical neck and proximal urethra. Abdominal pressure cannot open a normal urethra as the vesical neck and proximal urethra, 'the internal sphincter mechanism', are well supported intra-abdominally and not required to resist intra-abdominal pressure. In stress incontinence there is either an intermittent or complete failure of the urethral sphincter mechanism to effectively resist rises in abdominal pressure.

In women, sphincter abnormalities are of two types: urethral hypermobility and intrinsic sphincter deficiency (ISD). The two conditions may coexist. In the former condition, the urethral pressure is greater than the intravesical pressure. Sudden increases in intra-abdominal pressure cause unequal pressure transmissions so that the intravesical pressure is greater than the urethral pressure causing urine to leak. This unequal transmission of pressure occurs because rises in intra-abdominal pressure cause the poorly supported urethra to descend outside the abdominal cavity. Such patients have moderately high abdominal leak point pressure and respond well to operations aimed at restoring the anatomical defect, for example colposuspension.

Poor urethral closure or ISD is often encountered in female patients with myelodysplasia and after radical pelvic surgery. It is particularly common in patients who have failed multiple previous operations for stress incontinence. In these patients video urodynamic studies show that the bladder neck and proximal urethra are open at rest without detrusor contraction. The abdominal pressure required to cause urinary leakge, i.e. the abdominal leak pressure, is low. Surgical augmentations of urethral pressure by slings or implantation of artificial sphincter mechanisms are treatment options available. However, the increased urethral resistance that occurs may result in a parallel increase in detrusor compliance and pressure and subsequent upper-tract damage. These findings form the basis for the treatment of such patients with injectable materials. These materials are able to coapt the urethra and thereby resist abdominal pressure without a concomitant increase in voiding pressure and with no significant change in urethral resistance.[3] It has been suggested that it is not the urethral coaption that is important but the height of the submucosal humps produced by the injected material.[4]

In men, sphincter abnormalities are caused either by surgical trauma, most commonly following a prostatectomy or treatment of a urethral stricture. Neurological causes include spina bifida, thoracolumbar spinal abnormalities, anterior spinal artery syndrome and radical pelvic surgery (e.g. abdominoperineal resection). Treatment options here include an artificial sphincter or sling procedure or the periurethral injection of one of the materials currently available.

Injectable materials

Injectable materials were first used as a method of controlling urinary incontinence by Murless et al.[5] in 1938. They injected the sclerosing agent sodium morrhuate into the anterior vaginal wall so that the resulting scarring compressed the urethra. In 1955, Quackels described two successful cases where paraffin had been injected perineally.[6] Sachse[7] injected the sclerosant Dondren into the urethra with some success but this technique was complicated by the development of pulmonary emboli detected clinically and radiologically. The work of Arnold in 1962[8] using Polytef injections for vocal cord augmentation suggested its use as a material for the treatment of urinary incontinence. The urological application of Polytef was pioneered by Politano et al.[9,10] Since then, collagen, autologous fat and silicone have been used. Bioglass has been suggested as a possible alternative injectable. The use of these injectable materials has added a new dimension to the treatment of incontinence. The technique can be offered as a relatively simple day-case procedure and has potential not only as an effective treatment option but also in reducing the cost for treating incontinence.

Patient selection

The best candidates for treatment with injectable materials are those with intrinsic sphincter deficiency with good anatomical support and urodynamic or radiological evidence of failure of the proximal part of the urethra to close at rest in the absence of detrusor contraction. The easiest objective determinant is to measure leak point pressure, i.e. the intravesical pressure at which fluid instilled into the bladder escapes through the urethra. This should be done with the patient standing. In men, such investigations are not usually necessary. Incontinence demonstrated by coughing, straining or exercise is sufficient evidence that ISD is present. The measurement of leak pressure, if low, is supportive of ISD but can be unreliable in women with large cystocoeles. Urinary-tract infections must be treated as should detrusor instability. Patients with urethral hypermobility and high abdominal leak pressures are best treated by a suspension procedure, though where this fails injectable materials are indicated. Patients with combined urethral hypermobility and ISD are best treated initially by sling procedures. Patients with a known hypersensitivity to bovine collagen should be treated with an alternative injectable material.

Teflon

Polytetrafluoroethylene when pyrolysed becomes Polytef. Polytef paste for injection is sterile and contains a mixture of Polytef, glycerine and polysorbate. It has been used for vocal cord augmentation since 1962 and used initially by Politano et al. in 1974 in the treatment of post-prostatectomy incontinence and subsequently used for the treatment of women with stress incontinence.

Surgical technique

Women
The original technique described by Politano involved preliminary cystoscopy and urethral calibration to exclude a stricture. A 4-in. long 17 gauge needle was inserted via the perineum and advanced periurethrally

toward the bladder neck, the urethra being visualized endoscopically. Submucosal injections are given in the 3, 6, 9 and 12 o'clock positions using a total volume of 10–14 ml. The procedure can also be carried out transurethrally using instruments designed by Storz and Wolf.[11] Broad-spectrum antibiotics are given immediately prior to the procedure and continued for one week after.

Men

Broad-spectrum antibiotics are given prior to the procedure and continued for one week. The injections were initially given via the perineum but since 1984 the injections are performed transurethrally under direct vision using instruments designed by Storz and Wolf.[12] The Polytef is injected submucosally into the area corresponding to the external sphincter or just distal to it in the 3, 6, 9 and 12 o'clock positions to close the urethral channel. A 12 French Foley catheter is inserted or a suprapubic cystotomy performed. A trial of voiding is carried out the following day.

Results

Women

Lopez et al. 1993[11] reported on 128 women treated between 1964 and 1991. Sixty percent had undergone previous surgical treatment for incontinence. The mean follow-up was 31 months (range 21–63 months). An excellent result was defined as completely continent and occurred in 70 patients (54.7%) and a good result, defined as an improvement with need for minimal protection, occurred in 23 patients (18%). Thirty-five patients (27%) failed. Patients most likely to fail included those with periurethral fibrosis secondary to previous surgery and those with an unstable bladder. A Kaplan Meier analysis suggested that the probability of continence at 1, 5 and 10 years was 0.815, 0.605 and 0.454, respectively. Other authors have not been able to report such results. Lotenfoe et al. 1993[13] using a modified injection technique in 18 patients reported a cure rate of 39%, improvement of 17% and failure of 44%. Of 26 women reported by Beckingham et al. 1992,[14] at one month 15% were completely dry and 80% noted improvement. However, at 3 years only 27% were improved and 7% were dry. Lim et al. in 1983[15] showed an initial improvement in 54% of 28 women but only 21% remained improved at one year. Exclusion of patients with detrusor instability increased their success rate to 70% (30% cured). Long-term follow-up studies by Buckley et al. in 1994[16] also reported a reduction in success rate over time. Studying 58 women with stress incontinence, early follow-up at 3 months to one year showed 38 patients (60%) were dry or had an improvement of symptoms but on longer follow-up (mean 49 months) only 38% were dry or improved. Patients who are not improved can have further injections. However, in this study following two injections, 17 of 19 patients remained wet, and following three treatments three of four patients remained wet. Three patients developed retention, as a result of granuloma balls and one patient developed chronic retention due to bladder neck fibrosis. Six patients developed a rigid fibrotic or drainpipe urethra as a result of the injections. Three of six had had no previous surgery.

Men

Politano has treated 720 men who were incontinent for at least one year following prostatectomy:[17] the average number of injections per patient was 1.4 and the average volume of Polytef paste per injection 18 ml; 400 patients were incontinent following a transurethral resection; 312 were cured and 40 improved; 50% of the failures had received only one injection; 172 were incontinent following an open prostatectomy; 96 were cured, 32 improved and 44 failed; 18 of the 44 failures had received only one injection; 148 patients were incontinent following a radical prostatectomy, of whom 64 were cured, 36 improved and 48 failed; 16 of the 48 failures had received only one injection. Unfortunately the author does not provide details of long-term follow-up.

Complications

Mild dysuria, frequency and perianal discomfort occurs in most patients but usually resolves in 2 to 3 weeks. The lack of long-term success, technical difficulties with the procedure, the need for repeat injections and reports of submucosal extrusion of paste, granuloma formation and migration of particles to lymph nodes, lung and brain have limited the acceptability of its use. The longest clinical experience using Teflon is that of Lopez et al.[11] Until there are more long-term studies and the clinical significance of particle migration and local tissue response is established, the use of Teflon for incontinence should be limited to the elderly. The disadvantages associated with Teflon have led to the development of alternative materials that aim to combine high rates of success with minimal local and distant tissue reaction.

Collagen (Contigen)

This is a sterile non-pyrogenic purified form of bovine dermal collagen, cross-linked with glutaraldehyde and dispersed in a phosphate-buffered physiological saline. Cross-linking of bovine collagen aims to increase durability and decrease the potential for local immune reactions. The fear of development of an autoimmune response to human collagen following injection of bovine collagen has not been shown. However, as it is a foreign protein and potentially allergenic, skin testing must be performed 30 days before treatment. In a multicentre study, only 11 of 427 patients who were tested demonstrated this hypersensitivity.[18] Contigen begins to degrade in 12 weeks and is completely degraded in 9–19 months. Booster injections are therefore required in the majority of patients.

Surgical technique

Men

The injection can be performed either through a needle placed directly through a cystoscope or periurethrally with a spinal needle inserted percutaneously and observing the position of the needle cystoscopically. The Contigen delivery system consists of a 3-ml LuerLok syringe containing 2.5 ml of glutaraldehyde cross-linked collagen in its buffered solution. This is attached to a 5 French thermoplastic catheter with a 1.5-cm 20 gauge needle. The injection is made under direct vision under the urothelium. Three or four injections are made with the bevel of the needle facing the urethral lumen. The injection should be placed immediately above the external sphincter. Sufficient collagen should be injected under the urethral mucosa to occlude the urethral lumen. The technique of suburothelial injection has a significant learning curve and extravasation of the Contigen into the urethral lumen is not uncommon but does not appear to be harmful. Should significant extravasation occur from a number of the injection sites, then the procedure is best abandoned and repeated a few weeks later.

Women

Though the same technique can be used as in men, the author's present preference is to use a periurethral injection under direct vision using a 17 French cystoscope with a 0° lens. The injection is given through a 22 gauge spinal needle, the needle being inserted with the obturator in position and the bevel of the needle facing the urethral lumen. Injections given in the 3, 6 and 9 o'clock positions immediately proximal to the bladder neck are usually sufficient to close the urethral lumen.

The procedure in both men and women can be performed under local anaesthesia using lidocaine gel into the urethra and plain lignocaine injections periurethrally. This technique has the advantage of being able to test immediately the appropriateness of the Contigen injection. The patient can be asked to stand and carry out procedures to increase intra-abdominal pressure. Should urine leakage persist, further injections of Contigen can be given. Should the patient be unable to void postinjection, self-catheterization with a 10 French urethral catheter should be instituted.

Broad-spectrum antimicrobials should be administered immediately prior to the injection treatment and for 5 days following.

Results

In a series of 134 men with intrinsic sphincter deficiency followed up for more than one year, only 22 were dry though 70 were better; 42 had no improvement. In the same study, 137 females with ISD were treated, 63 of whom were dry and 47 better, with no improvement in 27. Of interest, 8 of 17 women with hypermobility were also dry. Seventeen patients with incontinence following radiotherapy (the authors do not state as to where the radiotherapy was given) were also treated. Two patients were dry and 8 better.[3]

In a study of 119 females with urethral incontinence of whom 86 had had previous incontinence surgery, 42 were cured and 57 improved. The 42 cured patients required a mean of 6.6 ml of collagen given over 1.8 treatments and have been followed for a mean of 11 months. The 57 improved patients required a mean of 12.7 ml given in three treatments and have been followed for 7 months. The incontinence in this group of patients was classified by radiological types 1, 2 and 3. Each radiological group responded equally well to the collagen injection[19]. In a study of 17 patients, which included 16 men and one woman,[20] 6 of the 16 men were incontinent following a transurethral prostatectomy or bladder-neck resection and the remaining 10 incontinent from a radical prostectomy. Follow-up ranged from 9 to 23 months after the last injection. Three men were cured or greatly improved and 5 were improved, 6 unchanged and 1 was worse.

Long-term results of collagen injections are still required. Short-term results show that they are safe and effective though the majority of patients will require more than one injection.

Bioglass

Bioglass is a bioactive glass composed of calcium oxide, calcium silicone and sodium oxide. It binds to tissues with minimal inflammatory response by attachment of collagen to its surface.[21] To date, there have been no reports of toxicity in animal studies[22] but it has not yet been adequately tested in humans for the treatment of incontinence.

Autologous fat

Autologous fat has the advantage over other injectable materials as it is readily available, easily obtainable, biocompatible and inexpensive. There is no risk of allergic reaction, nor any worry regarding migration or carcinogenicity. First reports of its use in the treatment of urinary incontinence in females appeared in 1989.[23,24]

Surgical technique[25]

The subcutaneous tissues of the lower abdominal wall are anaesthetized with 5 ml of 0.5% lignocaine. A 60-ml syringe containing 1 ml of saline attached to a 16-gauge needle is passed into the anaesthetized subcutaneous area between the index finger and the thumb. Traction is placed on the plunger of the syringe, exerting a negative pressure. The needle is moved backwards and forwards in a radial direction. Approximately 15 ml of fat are removed. It may be necessary to insert the needle in two or three different areas to obtain this volume. The syringe is then filled with saline, the fat rising to the surface, so that the excess saline can then be removed. The urethra is anaesthetized with lignocaine gel and 2% lignocaine injected at the 3 o'clock and 9 o'clock positions on either side of the urethra. A cystoscope is passed and the syringe and needle containing the fat are passed alongside the urethra with the bevel of the needle facing the urethral lumen. The fat is injected under the urethral mucosa. The procedure is repeated on the other side to cause complete coaption.

Results

Women with hypermobility and men with postprostatectomy incontinence derived no significant benefit from this treatment. Of 12 women with ISD, 10 (83%) were improved at one month and of the 9 who continued treatment, 7 underwent 14 injections (mean 2.4) during the follow-up which ranged from 12 to 30 months. All patients had some degree of subjective and objective improvement for at least one year following the last injection of autologous fat.[25] A further study of 15 women with stress incontinence and 5 men with postadenomectomy incontinence followed for at least one year showed good results in 23% of the cases with stress incontinence but none of the incontinent patients postprostatectomy benefited.[26]

Complications

The main disadvantage of fat is the variability of reabsorption and the degree of eventual connective-tissue replacement. Most studies report a 10–20% survival rate of fat. Bartynski et al. using a rabbit ear model to track histological events after fat injection reported final viability of 20–30%.[27] As a result, repeated injections are often necessary and the results unpredictable. Further trials are required to assess both the short- and long-term benefits of fat injection.

Macroplastique™

This is the most recently developed of the injectable materials. Macroplastique™ implants are sterile solid textured polydimethylsiloxane (silicone rubber) particles suspended in a non-silicone carrier gel. They are designed to act as a bulking agent. The non-silicone carrier gel consists of polyvinylpyrrolidone which is removed by the reticuloendothelial system and excreted unchanged (not metabolized) through the kidneys. The silicone rubber particles becoming capsulated in fibrin and with time collagen formation occurs. The manufacturers, Uroplasty Incorporated, now acknowledge that at least 25% of the particles have a diameter of $\leqslant 50\,\mu m$, though the majority are in the range 100–300 μm.[28]

Surgical technique

Preoperative antibiotics are given and continued for 5 days post-operatively. Although the procedure can be performed under a local or a general anaesthetic, a local anaesthetic is preferred as further injections can be given if the initial response is not satisfactory. The author prefers to pass the needle through a nephroscope, the inside of the needle needs to be lubricated and the Macroplastique™ injected submucosally with the aid of a rachet syringe (Fig. 3.1). Approximately 1.0–1.75 ml of Macro-plastique™ is injected at 3, 6 and 9 o'clock to produce mucosal coaption immediately proximal to the bladder neck.

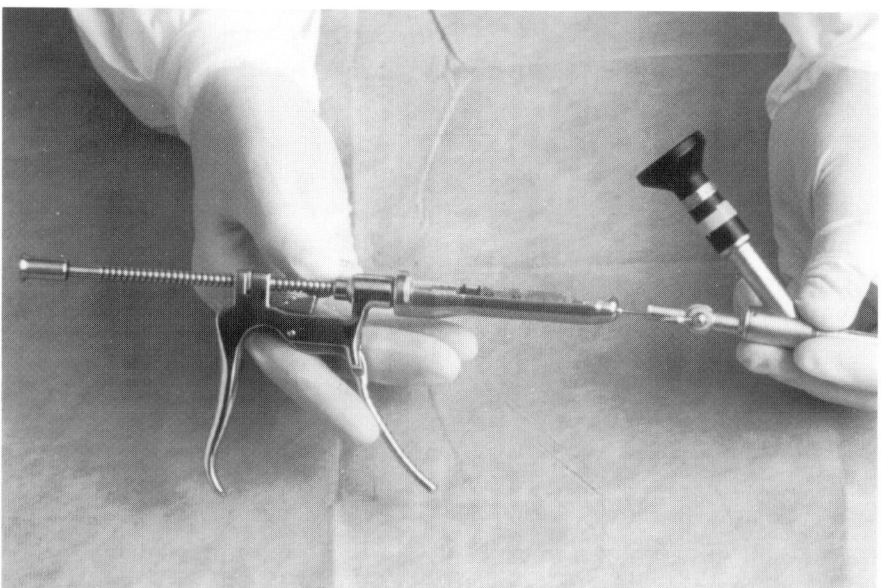

Fig. 3.1. The Macroplastique™ injection device.

Results

Buckley et al.[29] studied 144 patients with urodynamically proven stress incontinence. The procedure was performed as a day case and the average amount of Macroplastique™ injected was 4.4 ml. Patients were reviewed at 1, 3, 6 and 12 months. The follow-up range was 6–24 months with a mean of 17 months. One hundred of 144 patients were dry (70%), 14 were improved (10%) and 29 were wet (20%). Most failures occurred within three months of injection and the re-injection rate was 1.4. James et al.[30] treated 40 women with stress incontinence, confirmed on medium fill videocystometry. Fifteen had previously undergone incontinence surgery. Three months after a single injection, 16 (40%) were completely dry and 13 (33%) were improved. There were no failures later than 6 weeks. Twenty-three patients had been followed for one year and of these 16 (70%) remained completely dry. Twenty-one men with stress incontinence following transurethral resection received 31 injections of Macroplastique[TM]; 9 of the 21 patients are dry and 4 improved. The follow-up in this study was up to 24 months.[31] Glass and Henalla[32] report equal subjective benefits in 47 patients who were treated either by injections of Macroplastique or a Burch colposuspension. The complication rate and time in hospital was much higher in those receiving the Burch colposuspension. They recommend injections of Macroplastique[TM] as an effective and efficient alternative first-line treatment for the management of genuine incontinence.

Complications

Mild dysuria was common and a small proportion of patients developed retention of urine which rapidly resolved following periods of intermittent self-catheterization or the insertion of a small urethral catheter for 24 hours.

Conclusion

The use of injectable materials has added a new dimension to the treatment of urinary incontinence. It is most effective in the management of patients with intrinsic sphincter deficiency. It offers an attractive alternative to surgery, especially in the elderly and those unfit for major surgery, since it can be performed as a day-case procedure under local anaesthesia. As such, it has a potential to greatly reduce the cost of treatment of this very common condition. Injections with fat and collagen need to be repeated and long-term results of injection of Macroplastique[TM] with regard to safety are still required.

References

1. Bates P, Bradley WE, Glen E et al. The standardisation of terminology of lower urinary tract function. J Urol 1979; 121: 551–4
2. *Morbidity and Mortality Weekly Report.* Urinary incontinence among hosptitalized persons aged 65 years and older, United States 1984–87. U.S. Department of Health and Human Services, 1991; 40: 26
3. McGuire EJ, Appel RA. Transurethral collagen injection for urinary incontinence. Urology 1994; 43: 413–15

4. Khullar V, Cardoza LD, Abbott D et al. The mechanism of continence achieved with GAX collagen as determined by ultrasound. Neurourol Urodynam 1993; 12 Abstract 78: 439–40

5. Murless BC. The injection treatment of stress incontinence. J Obstet Gynaecol Br Empire 1938; 45: 67–73

6. Quackels R. Deux incontinences après adenomectomie guéries par injection de paraffine dans le périnée. Acta Urol Belg 1955; 23: 259–62

7. Sachse S. Treatment of urinary incontinence with sclerosing solutions. Indications, results, complications. Urol Int 1963; 15: 225–44

8. Artnold GE. Vocal rehabilitation of paralytic dysphonia. IX. Technique of intracordal injection. Arch Otolaryngol 1962; 76: 76–83

9. Politano VA, Small MP, Harper JM, Lynne CM. Periurethral Teflon injection for urinary incontinence. Trans Am Assoc Genitourin Surg 1973; 65: 54–7

10. Politano VA, Small MP, Harper JM, Lynne CM. Periurethral Teflon injection for urinary incontinence. J Urol 1974; 111: 180–3

11. Lopez AE, Padron OF, Patsias G, Politano VA. Transurethral polytetrafluoroethylene injection in female patients with urinary incontinence. J Urol 1993; 150: 856–8

12. Kaufman M, Lockhart JL, Silverstein MJ, Politano VA. Transurethral polytetrafluoroethylene injection for postprostatectomy urinary incontinence. J Urol 1984; 132: 463–4

13. Lotenfoe R, O'Kelly JK, Helal M, Lockhart JL. Periurethral polytetrafluoroethylene paste injection in incontinent female subjects: surgical indications and improved surgical technique. J Urol 1993; 149: 279–82

14. Beckingham IJ, Wemyss-Holden G, Lawrence WT. Long term follow up of women treated with periurethral Teflon injections for stress incontinence. Br J Urol 1992; 69: 580–3

15. Lim KB, Ball AJ, Feneley RCL. Periurethral Teflon injection: a simple treatment for urinary incontinence. Br J Urol 1983; 55: 208–10

16. Buckley JK, Lingam K, Meddings RN, Scott R. Injectable Teflon paste for female stress incontinence: Long term follow up and results. J Urol 1994; 151, Abstract 764, 418A

17. Politano VA. Transurethral Polytef injection for postprostatectomy urinary incontinence. Br J Urol 1992; 69: 26–8

18. Appell RA. Collagen injection therapy for urinary incontinence. Urol Clin N Am 1994; 21: 177–82

19. Herschorn S, Steele D, Radomski S. Intraurethral collagen for female stress incontinence. Neurourol Urodynam 1993; 12 Abstract 77: 437–8

20. Dairiki Shortliffe LM, Freiha FS, Kessler R et al. Treatment of urinary incontinence by the periurethral implantation of glutaraldehyde cross-linked collagen. J Urol 1989; 141: 538–41

21. Wilson J, Nolletti D. Bonding of soft tissues to Bioglass. In Yamamuro T, Hench LL, Wilson J (eds) Handbook of bioactive ceramics, bioactive glasses and glass ceramics. Boca Raton Florida, CRC Press. 1990, Vol. 1, 283

22. Dixon Walker R, Wilson K, Clark AE. Injectable Bioglass as a potential substitute for injectable polytetrafluoroethylene. J Urol 1992; 148: 645–7

23. Gonzalez-Garibay S, Jimeno C, York M et al. Endoscopic autotransplantation of fat tissue in the treatment of urinary incontinence in the female. J Urol (Paris) 1989; 95: 363–6

24. Santiago-Gonzalez de Garibay AM, Castro-Morrondo J, Castillo-Jimeno JM et al. Endoscopic injection of autologous adipose tissue in the treatment of female incontinence. Arch Esp Urol 1989; 42: 143–6

25. Santarosa RP, Blaivas JG. Periurethral injection of autologous fat for the treatment of sphincteric incontinence. J Urol 1994; 151: 607–11

26. Gonzalezde-Garibay AS, Castillo-Jimeno JM, Villanueva-Perez I et al. Treatment of urinary stress incontinence using paraurethral injection of autologous fat. Arch Esp Urol 1991; 44: 595–600

27. Bartynski J, Marion MS, Wang TD. Histopathologic evaluation of adipose autografts in a rabbit ear model. Otolaryngol Head Neck Surg 1990; 102: 314–21

28. Aaronson IA. Current status of the 'Sting'. An American perspective. Br J Urol 1995. 75: 121–5

29. Buckley JF, Lingam K, Meddings R et al. Injectable silicone macroparticles for female urinary incontinence. Presented at the Annual Meeting of BAUS, Harrogate, UK, 1993

30. James MJ, Iacovou JW, Lemberger RJ, Kockelbergh RC. A one year follow up of periurethral silicone for simple stress incontinence. Presented at the Annual Meeting of BAUS, Harrogate, UK, 1993
31. Buckley JF, Patterson PJ, Smith M et al. Injectable silicone macroparticles for postprostatectomy incontinence. Presented at the Annual Meeting of BAUS, Harrogate, UK, 1993
32. Glass K, Henalla SM. Macroplastique^{TM} implant versus Burch colposuspension in the treatment of genuine stress incontinence. Presented at the ICS 24th Annual Meeting, Prague, 1994

Biocompatibility and tolerability of urinary-tract implanted material (endoprostheses) and alloplastic material used for the regeneration or replacement of upper urinary tract

M. Ruutu   M. Talja   L. Cormio

Introduction: general definitions

Biocompatibility is defined as the ability of a material to perform with an appropriate host response in a specific application. Absolute biocompatibility means that the material does not cause any adverse effects on the host or vice versa. Such a situation is a utopian state of affairs which cannot be expected at present.[1] Alloplastic materials always cause a tissue reaction. The magnitude and the kind of reaction is dependent on the biomaterial and the specific properties of the tissue environment. The urinary tract is a special environment because the biomaterial is in contact with urine and the uroepithelium. A biomaterial is defined as a substance which interfaces with tissue at least at some stage of treatment. Biomaterials can be of natural or synthetic origin.

Urinary-tract endoprostheses

Urinary-tract endoprostheses can be used in the upper or lower urinary tract. Various stents are used in the ureter mostly to treat upper-tract obstruction or ureteric fistulas, or to bridge partial defects in the ureteric wall. Alloplastic tubes to replace a gap in the upper urinary tract have been tried with different materials, but these attempts have usually failed due to several reasons (see Chapter 5).

Urethral stents are used mainly to treat obstructive dysfunction of the lower urinary tract. The most usual clinical indications for a stent include benign prostatic hyperplasia, urethral stricture and neurogenic voiding dysfunction. Urethral stents are discussed in Chapter 6.

An endoprosthesis is usually more comfortable to the patient as compared with catheters communicating to the outer surface of the body, such as nephrostomy tubes or indwelling or suprapubic bladder catheters. The use of various endoprostheses, however, is associated with multiple problems depending on the physical and chemical properties of the prosthetic materials, the multiple tissue reactions and the effects of urine on the prosthesis itself.

Materials

Endoprostheses can be made of a variety of materials. The polymeric biomaterials currently used for ureteric stents include silicone and polyurethane and their derivates. The polymeric complex macromolecules are formed by linkage of monomeric chains. These macromolecules are versatile and thus suitable as endoprosthetic material. Biomaterials used for ureteric stents should have physical and chemical properties suitable for good performance and biocompatibility.

Investigations comparing materials used for ureteric stents have been extensively carried out by Mardis and co-workers.[2,3]

Low coefficient of friction is essential for easy insertion of the prosthesis. The coefficient of friction does not correlate with the roughness of the surface, as one would expect, as the clearly rough polyurethane surface has a lower coefficient than the clearly smooth silicone surface. Wettable materials, like hydrogel, have proved to have a lower coefficient of friction than the not-wettable ones. The use of hydrogel-coated stents and of hydrogel-coated guidewires has been recommended to facilitate stent insertion.

Radiopacity is essential for a correct placement of the stent. Attention should be paid to the chemicals used to achieve radiopacity, as Ramsey and co-workers[4] proved that the barium or bismuth used to make the stent radiopaque leached from the polymer and caused encrustation.

Memory, which is defined as the ability of the stent to assume the original coil or other intended form after removal of the straightening guidewire used for the application, is essential to prevent migration.

Tensile strength indicates the resistance of the biomaterial against breakage. In investigations comparing materials for ureteric stents, tensile strength of various 6 F ureteric stents was highest in stents made of polyurethane or Silitek[R] (a proprietary silicone-based block copolymer). It was lowest in a pure silicone stent, and C-Flex[R] (a proprietary silicone-modified styrene/ethylene/butylene block copolymer) gave intermediate values. An important finding was that the stents invariably broke across the sideholes. It has earlier been shown that the sideholes give considerable drainage advantage. In a model, flow rate in stents with sideholes was usually twice the flow rate in identical stents without sideholes.[5]

The internal/external diameter ratio should be as low as possible in order to allow for optimal flow conditions inside and around the stent. The internal/external diameter ratio depends on the stent material. The ratio was shown to be highest in Percuflex[R] stents (a proprietary olefinic block copolymer) and also over 0.5 in polyurethane and C-Flex[R] stents. Pure silicone stents from different manufacturers had a lower ratio (<0.5).[3] A large internal diameter is of advantage, but urinary flow is known to occur also around the endoprosthesis.[6,7]

Chemical inertness, which means that the biomaterial should not cause deleterious effects either on the urothelium, in terms of epithelial destruction and inflammatory changes, or on urine, in terms of encrustation, stone formation and infection, is an essential prerequisite for biomaterials.

Hydrodynamics of the upper urinary tract associated with indwelling ureteric stents

In vitro pressure–flow studies have shown that ureteric stents can convey supraphysiologic flow rates with low pressures.[5–8] In the clinical situation, the stents cannot always accommodate a normal urine flow. Urine flow occurs also around the stent.[7,9,10]

Renal pelvic pressure measurements in experimental animals show increased pressures in the acute stage of ureteric intubation. This phenomenon is dependent on an open tube flow, where a standing column of urine causes direct transmission of pressure from the bladder to the renal pelvis.[11,12] Over a few weeks, the ureter adapts to the endoprosthesis, and the renal pelvic pressure declines while the ureter dilates and urine flow becomes increasingly extraluminal despite patency of the stent.[7,12,13] Our recent investigations in pigs have shown that in some cases a high-pressure condition can persist for at least 6 weeks after ureteric intubation, and in growing animals, also renal parenchymal reduction may occur.[14] Prolonged stenting (>3 weeks) was likewise seen to lead to loss of renal function in 2 of 18 renal units of male rabbits, due to severe hydronephrosis or infection.[15] In rabbits there was similarly a positive correlation between renal obstruction and long-term ureteric stenting.[16]

Pressure–flow investigations in patients with indwelling double-J stent and nephrostomy tube showed that proper drainage of the bladder occurred in 17 of 20 patients when average renal pressure was 19.9 cmH$_2$O.[8] Normal intrapelvic pressure is less than 10 cmH$_2$O and rises up to 25 cmH$_2$O during a peristaltic wave. The majority of the investigated patients had extrinsic ureteric obstruction. A simultaneous in vitro experiment mimicking extrinsic obstruction by creating pressure on the stents or kinking them showed that hard polyurethane stents tolerated compression and kinking reasonably well without remarkable alterations in their flow characteristics. Compression caused diminution in the flow rate of a soft silicone stent, and flow nearly ceased as the result of kinking of the stent.

In Cormio's experiment,[14] all the renal units (29% of the stented units) showing significant parenchymal reduction were intubated with pure polyurethane stents. Polyurethane is a relatively hard material of high tensile strength. Stents made of pure polyurethane tolerate multiple sideholes without risk of breaking and can therefore be regarded as having an advantageous flow capacity. Yet they caused more hydrodynamic side effects on the upper tract, which speaks for the importance of the extraluminal drainage. Such drainage could be thought to be more readily possible in connection to softer stents.

Vesicoureteric or vesicorenal reflux of various grades occurs in connection to indwelling double-J stents. In the majority of patients it is of low grade during bladder filling and of high grade during voiding.[17]

Some patients experience flank pain during voiding, which could be due to reflux.[18] In experimental animals, bladder drainage during diuretic stress causes a significant decrease in intrapelvic pressure,[19] which is in agreement with the open-tube flow theory. The renal parenchymal reduction seen in some growing animals could thus be due to a reflux phenomenon or high intrapelvic pressure or the combination of both. Conversely, Culkin and coworkers[20] could not detect deterioration of renal function with DTPA renal scans in female canines with unilateral ureteric Surgitek® stents, despite vesicoureteric reflux and dilation of the stented ureter.

It is, however, evident that ureteric stents cause at least temporary upper-tract obstruction. They also cause vesicoureteric/vesicorenal reflux which may persist for as long as the stent is indwelling. Due to these hydrodynamic alterations, the indications for ureteric stenting should be considered carefully.

Effects of the stents on the ureteric wall

Indwelling ureteric stents are used for a variety of conditions, and thus remain in situ for time periods ranging from a few days to several months. The stent material is in close contact with the uroepithelium. There are only a few investigations of the effects of various modern stent materials on the wall of the ureter. The first authors to describe alloplastic materials in experimental ureteric surgery were Drake and co-workers in 1962.[21] Marked changes consisting of urothelial ulcerations, inflammatory infiltration and subepithelial fibroplasia, as well as smooth-muscle hypertrophy, were caused by latex and red rubber stents. Further studies have confirmed that latex causes severe changes in the uroepithelium. Most of these studies have focused on the urethra. It has been well documented in clinical series[22–24] and experimental studies[25] that toxic chemicals added to the latex base during the manufacturing process can leach out from the devices in situ causing severe chemical urethritis and stricture formation as a consequence. This deleterious effect is accentuated by low blood-flow conditions in the urethra, like extracorporeal perfusion during cardiac surgery, hypovolemic shock and arteriosclerosis.[26,27] In vitro cell-culture tests also document the toxicity of latex catheters.[25,28]

As material, latex is elastic, but the inner/outer diameter ratio of latex tubes is poor because of the thickness of the tube walls. The surface characteristics are rough, and latex is prone to encrustation. For all these reasons, latex has been abandoned in the manufacture of ureteric stents, but is still used in some tubes communicating to the outer surface of the body, such as urethral catheters, Malecot tubes and T tubes.

Silicone and other polymeric stents are also known to cause changes in the ureteric epithelium, but literature regarding such information is scarce. Ramsay and co-workers[4] took endoscopic cup biopsies from four ureters and 20 ureteric orifices of 24 patients whose ureters had been intubated with silicone or other polymer double-J stents. The biopsies were taken at the time of stent removal. The indwelling time ranged from 5 days to 6 months. Mucous metaplasia was seen in 12 (50%) biopsies and 10 of these biopsies were retrieved from stone-forming patients.

More detailed findings have been seen in animal experiments. In porcine ureters intubated with polyurethane stents, histological findings showed a constant and generalized thickening of the ureteric wall, and epithelial changes consisting of vacuolation of cells, patchy atrophy and hyperplasia.[7] Such epithelial changes were regarded as characteristic of excessive mucus production which also could provoke stent blocking. In a dog model,[29] silicone, C-Flex and polyurethane stents all caused a mild degree of ureteric oedema, but Silitek stents caused a fairly marked oedema. All polyurethane stents induced epithelial erosions and ulcerations, and the changes were often severe. The other stents rarely caused such changes. The authors concluded that the epithelial injury caused by polyurethane could be related to the irregularity of the material surface and to its hydrophobic character, and regarded silicone and C-Flex more suitable for ureteric stenting.

In a recent experiment, the influence of eight stent brands on porcine ureters was investigated both by histological and scanning electron microscopic (SEM) analysis after six weeks' intubation.[30] The findings were divided into two groups according to the biological characteristics of the lesions, i.e. superficial epithelial destruction and ureteric reactive changes. The histological and SEM scores were added up. Hydro-Plus (hydrogel-coated C-Flex) and silicone stents caused the mildest superficial destruction while polyurethane and C-Flex gave the highest scores (Table 4.1). Silicone and Sof-Flex had the lowest scores for reactive changes, while C-Flex had the highest. Representative electron microscopic samples from the different findings are seen in Figs 4.1 to 4.4. All stent brands were

Item	Superficial epithelial destruction	Ureteral reactive change
Controls	0	0
Silicone	0.9	0.4
Hydro-Plus	0.3	1.3
Sof-Flex	1.0	0.7
Blue	0.8	1.0
Grey	1.1	1.2
Puroflex	1.2	1.3
Polyurethane	1.4	1.3
C-Flex	1.4	1.6

Table 4.1. Scanning electron microscopy and histological analysis of porcine ureters and scanning electron microscopic analysis of various double-J stents after 6 weeks of intubation

Grade 0 = no change; Grade 1 = mild change; Grade 2 = moderate change; Grade 3 = severe change

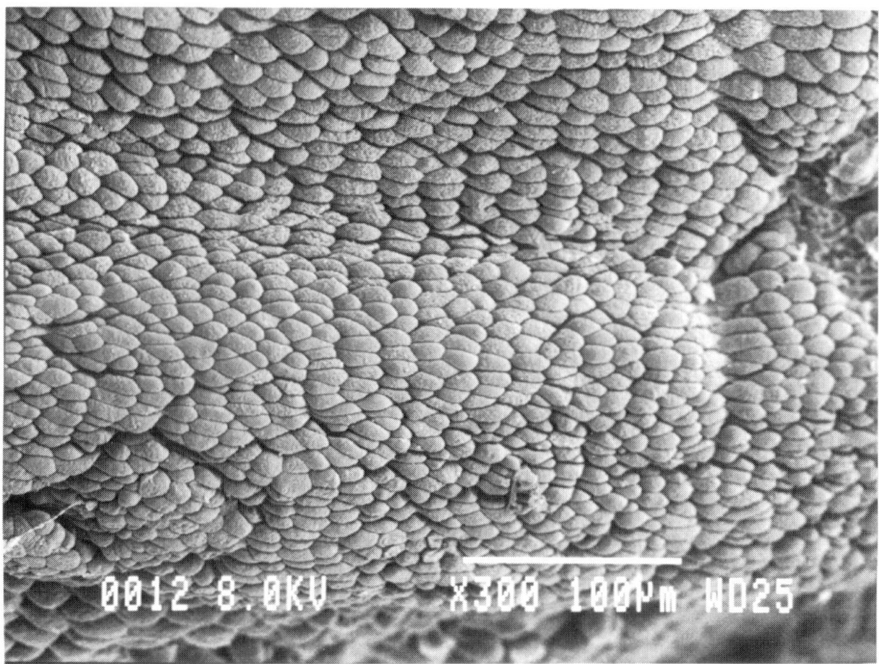

Fig. 4.1. Normal porcine ureteric epithelium.

analysed for cytotoxicity in a cell-culture model used in our earlier studies of urethral catheters.[25] The double-J stent brands made of modified polyurethane were cytotoxic but considerably less so than the latex catheter used as a toxic control sample. Other stent brands did not show any cytotoxicity. The cytotoxicity in vitro did not, however, correlate with the in vivo epithelial findings.

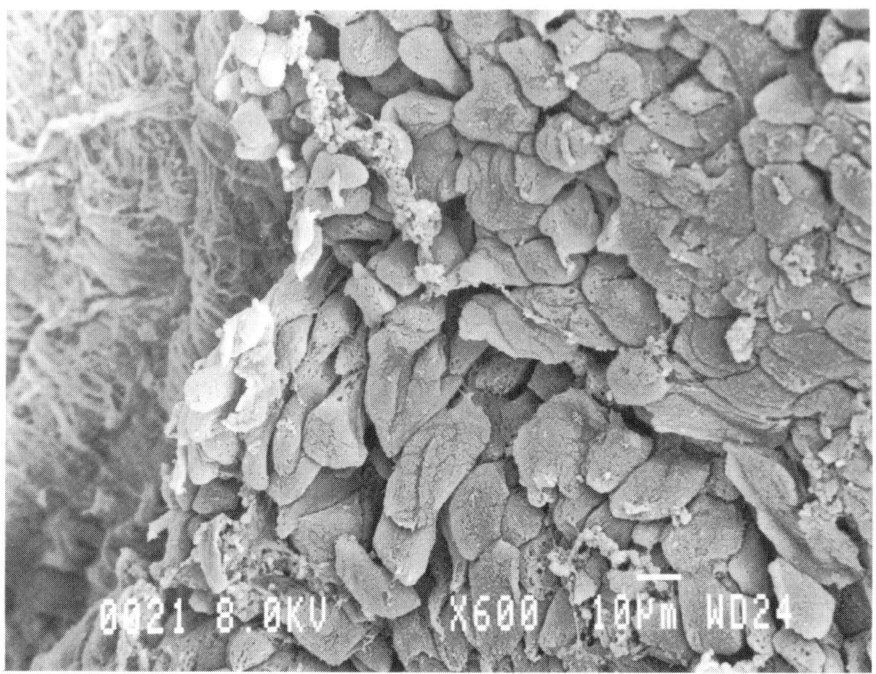

Fig. 4.2. Ureteric epithelium after six weeks' intubation with a polyurethane stent. Destructive changes (injured epithelial cells and loss of epithelium) are seen.

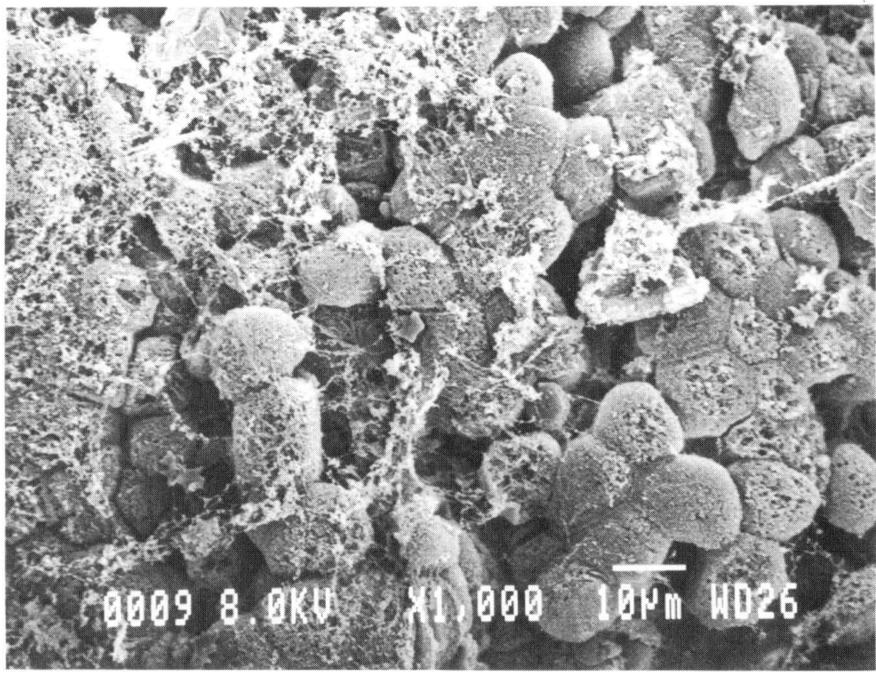

Fig. 4.3. Inflammatory reactive changes (accumulation of debris) caused by a C-Flex stent.

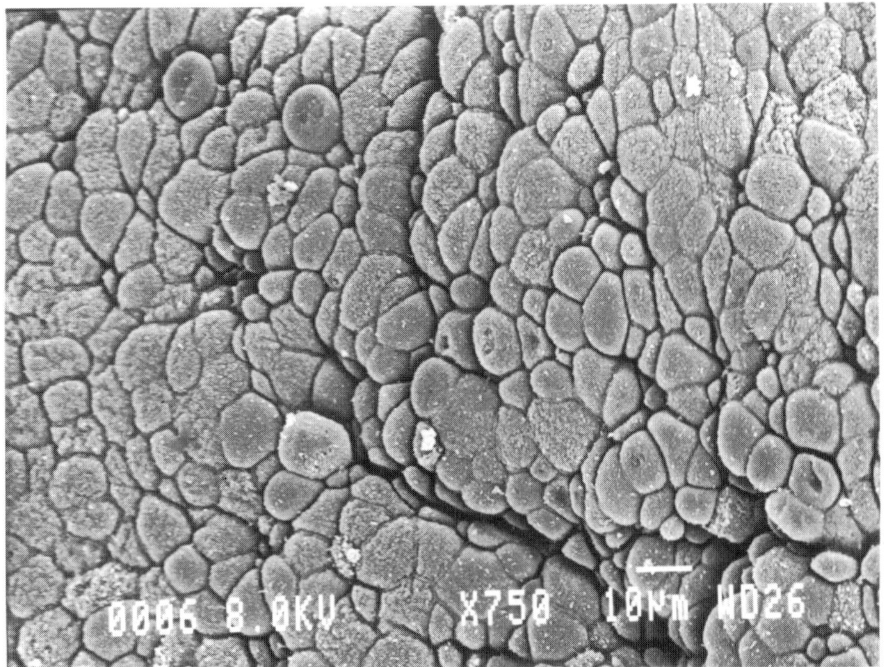

Fig. 4.4. Ureteric epithelium after six weeks' intubation with a Hydro-Plus stent. The epithelium looks almost similar to the control (Fig. 4.1).

Direct comparison of all findings of these different in vivo experiments is not possible, but there are some common features. Pure polyurethane stents caused histological lesions of a similar character in all three studies and gave high scores for epithelial injury in the two studies with a grading system.[29,30] Pure polyurethane was, however, not toxic in the cell-culture test, while stents made of modified polyurethane were. It could be thought that plasticizers used in the manufacture of modified softened polyurethane are responsible for the cytotoxicity. This cytotoxicity seems not to be clinically relevant in the ureter where blood circulation is normal and there is continuous extraluminal urine flow wiping out the leachable chemicals. It is not known whether cytotoxicity would be accentuated in ureters where circulation can be compromised, such as after radiotherapy or surgical trauma.

The urothelial changes following intubation with pure polyurethane stents are thus not dependent on cytotoxicity but on other factors. Polyurethane is stiff and has a high tensile strength and friction coefficient.[31] Such material properties may cause more hydrodynamic alterations and ureteric dilation and reaction in the ureteric wall than smooth materials with low friction coefficient. Polyurethane is also hydrophobic.[32] Hydrogel-coated stents are new products. Hydrogels are special hydrophilic polymers which swell on contact with water and retain water in the polymeric structure, thus making the material soft, flexible and slippery.[33] The coefficient of friction of hydrogel-coated catheters is lower than that of silicone catheters.[34] Hydrogel-coated latex catheters also showed smaller toxicity scores in dog urethra than silicone catheters.[35] The hydrogel coating seemed to protect diffusion of harmful products from the latex core, because scanning electron microscopic studies have shown that hydrogel coating remains mostly intact in use.[36] It is logical to assume that a hydrogel coating behaves in a similar way in the ureter as in the urethra, and the recent results of the high biocompatibility of hydrogel-coated ureteric stents[30] are in agreement with this hypothesis.

Encrustation and stone formation

The phenomenon of encrustation and stone formation on bladder catheters has been known as long as indwelling catheters have been used. This phenomenon appears in connection with urea-splitting organisms raising urinary pH and precipitating struvite.[37] The morphology of the mineral deposits has been studied in detail by scanning electron microscopy.[38] Hydrogel coating makes the catheter surface smooth and the furrows shallow.[36] Catheters coated with modified hydrogel or silicone elastomer, or pure silicone catheters, showed no statistical difference in their ability to resist encrustation in an in vitro model.[39] In a clinical series, hydrogel-coated catheters were less prone to encrustation than full silicone or siliconized latex catheters.[40] Hydrogel-coated urinary catheters are now generally recommended for long-term use in bladder catheterization.

Encrustation can also form on internal ureteric stents irrespective of whether there is bacterial urinary infection or not. The major risk factor for stent encrustation seems to be the stone-forming tendency of the patient.[9,41] Ramsay and co-workers[4] noted that 68% of stents were blocked at the time of removal after an indwelling period of 5 days up to 6 months. Mucous metaplasia was noted principally in stone-forming patients. Calcareous deposits on stents were already noted at two weeks, and encrustation increased with indwelling time. Silicone and polymer stents were blocked as easily, but the sample size was small. Recently, an experimental study in pigs confirmed that hydrogel-coated ureteric stents were less prone to encrustation than silicone stents.[30]

Encrustation is one of the major reasons for the failure of alloplastic urinary-tract replacement. The new polymeric biomaterials used in ureteric devices are not free from encrustation either. Hydrogel-coated ureteric stents may offer an advantage over stents with higher friction of coefficient. It remains to be seen whether these new stents can resist encrustation also in stone-forming patients.

Holmes and co-workers[42] have developed an encrustation model to provide a reproducible and quantitative assessment of the susceptibility of polymers to encrustation. In this model, a constant passage of sterile human urine over a polymer surface is used. Incorporation of fluorine-containing components in copolymers increased resistance to encrustation. Such reproducible tests are welcome for the development of new biomaterials.

Bacterial adherence and infection

It has been known for decades that bacteria in natural aquatic populations have a marked tendency to interact with surfaces.[43] Bacteria will adhere to a surface using exopolysaccharide glycocalyx polymers. Extensive bacterial biofilms have been found on a large number of medical devices made of a variety of biomaterials.[44] There is not a uniform correlation between biofilm formation and clinical infection. The role of antibiotic therapy remains unclear because bacteria in biofilms are not killed by antibiotics.[45] Thus a bacterial biofilm may form a constant nidus for infection, although a clinically evident infection can usually be treated by antibiotic therapy.[44] Keane and co-workers[41] found a profuse biofilm on 11 (28%) polyurethane ureteric stents removed from 40 patients. Bacteriuria with organisms isolated from the stents was seen in only three cases. There was no correlation between biofilm formation and stent encrustation. The authors concluded that ureteric stents are readily colonized by bacteria in vivo despite the use of peroperative antibiotic. Likewise, Reid and co-workers[46] found adherent pathogens on 27 of 30 (90%) ureteric stents. In half of these, the bacteria were present in low numbers but on the other stents, small or large microcolony biofilms were seen. Urine culture was positive in only 27% of the patients with colonized stents.

We have recently studied bacterial adhesion and biofilm formation on various indwelling double-J stents in vivo and in vitro to determine whether they could depend on the stent material. After 6 weeks of intubation in pig ureters, adherent bacteria were found on 9 of the 23 (39%) indwelling ureteric stents but only 2 of the 23 (9%) stents presented bacterial biofilms, i.e. several adherent bacteria surrounded by amorphous glycocalyx matrices. Significantly, urine culture was positive only in the two renal units intubated with the stents presenting bacterial biofilms, i.e. one Cook polyurethane stent and one Angiomed blue stent, suggesting that urinary infection develops in the presence of significant bacterial biofilm formation.

In the in vitro assay, only 1/1000–1/10 000 of the bacterial population, i.e. 0.1–0.01% of the bacterial inoculum, adhered to the stents. There was no statistically significant difference in bacterial adherence onto the various stent materials, pointing out that the properties of the various test materials did not influence bacterial adhesion. Conversely, we found a statistically significant difference in adhesion among the bacterial test strains, as one strain of E. coli adhered much more than the other test strains. Thus, bacterial adhesion onto biomaterials used for ureteric stents may depend on the properties of the bacteria rather than on those of the biomaterials.

The clinical significance of bacterial adherence to ureteric stents, and whether antimicrobial treatment is of any use, still remains unsolved. If antibiotics are used, it should be remembered that the most usual pathogens isolated from the biofilms are Gram-positive cocci.[41,46]

Biological tests for medical devices made of polymers

There are multiple tests which can be applied in the toxicity testing of medical devices. Urinary-tract endoprostheses belong to the category of surface devices in contact with mucous membranes and can be regarded as long-term devices (contact with body > 30 days). The recommendations for biological tests for such devices given by the International Standards Organization[47] are presented in Table 4.2.

Toxicity tests can be done in vivo or in vitro. In vitro cell-culture tests

Cytotoxicity
Sensitization assay
Irritation or intracutaneous reactivity
Subchronic toxicity
Genotoxicity

Table 4.2. Test panel for biomaterials of polymers category: surface devices/mucosal membranes. Contact > 30 days

are now regarded as the first-line screening tests, and the British Standards Institution has recently included a cell-culture test in the requirements of testing for biological hazards of urinary catheters.[48] Different animal tests are favoured by the manufacturers, and the rabbit muscle implantation test (United States Pharmacopeia) is the one most commonly used.[49]

Agreement between some cell-culture and animal test models has been reported.[28,50] Cell-culture tests are more sensitive, quantitative, simple and easily reproducible.[51] There are, however, problems in the interpretation of the results as to the biological hazard. Isolated cells lack the normal body environment, which may be protective against extrinsic toxins. Chemicals can affect several steps in the cell cycle, and different cell culture tests may give divergent results. Therefore, we have earlier recommended that catheters should not show any toxicity in a cell-culture test which is performed with a 100% catheter eluate.[52]

Ureteric stents made of modified polyurethane did not meet these criteria in our experiments.[30] Such toxicity limits may be too strict.

There exist no separate standards for ureteric stents or respective devices so far, but they can be discussed in the same category as urethral catheters as to their biological safety. Standardization work has to be continued to find reproducible and reliable biological tests for medical devices.

References

1. Williams DF. Biomaterials and biocompatibility: an introduction. In Williams DF (ed) Fundamental aspects of biocompatibility. Boca Raton, CRC Press, 1981; 1: 2–7
2. Mardis HK, Kroeger RM. Ureteral stents. Materials. Urol Clin N Am 1988; 15: 471–9
3. Mardis HK, Kroeger RM, Morton JJ, Donovan JM. Comparative evaluation of materials used for internal ureteral stents. J Endourol 1993; 7: 105–15
4. Ramsay JWA, Crocker RP, Bell AJ et al. Urothelial reaction to ureteric intubation. A clinical study. Br J Urol 1987; 60: 504–5
5. Mardis HK, Kroeger RM, Hepperlen TW et al. Polyethylene double-pigtail ureteral stents. Urol Clin N Am 1982; 9: 95–101
6. Griffiths OJ. The mechanisms of urine transport in the upper urinary tract. 2. The discharge of the bolus into the bladder and dynamics at high rates of flow. Neurourol Urodynam 1983; 2: 167–70
7. Ramsay JWA, Payne SR, Gosling PT et al. The effects of double J stenting on unobstructed ureters. An experimental and clinical study. Br J Urol 1985; 57: 630–4
8. Hubner WA, Plas EG, Stoller ML. The double-J ureteral stent: in vivo and in vitro flow studies. J Urol 1992; 148: 278–80
9. Finney RP. Double J and diversion stents. Urol Clin N Am 1982; 9: 89–94
10. Shabsigh R, Gleeson MJ, Griffith DP. The benefits of stenting on a more-or-less routine basis prior to extracorporeal shock-wave lithotripsy. Urol Clin N Am 1988; 15: 493–7
11. Tofft HP, Frokaier J, Djurhuus JC. Renal pelvic peristalis in pigs during standardized flow rate variations. Urol Int 1986; 41: 292–8
12. Payne SR, Ramsay JWA. The effects of double J stents on renal pelvic dynamics in the pig. J Urol 1988; 140: 637–41
13. Roos R, Lykoudis PS. The fluid mechanics of the ureter with an inserted catheter. J Fluid Mech 1971; 46: 265–71
14. Cormio L, Koivusalo A, Mäkisalo H et al. The effects of various indwelling JJ stents on renal pelvic pressure and renal parenchymal thickness in the pig. Br J Urol 1994; 74: 440–3
15. el-Deen ME, Khalaf I, Rahim FA. Effect of internal ureteral stenting of normal ureter on the upper urinary tract: an experimental study. J Endourol 1993; 7(5): 399–405
16. Galal H, Lazica A, Lampel A, el-Guiochi F et al. Management of ureteral strictures by different modalities and effect of stents on upper tract drainage. J Endourol 1993; 7(5): 411–17
17. Mosli HA, Farsi HMLA, Al-Zimaity MF et al. Vesicoureteral reflux in patients with double pigtail stents. J Urol 1991; 146: 966–9
18. Bregg K, Riehle RA Jr. Morbidity associated with indwelling internal ureteral stents after shock wave lithotripsy. J Urol 1989; 141: 510–12
19. Payne SR, Ramsay JWA. The effects of double J stents on renal pelvic dynamics in the pig. J Urol 1988; 140: 637–41
20. Culkin DJ, Zitman R, Bundrick WS et al. Anatomic, functional and pathologic changes from internal ureteral stent placement. Urology 1992; 40: 385–90
21. Drake WM, Carroll J, Bartone F et al. Evaluation of materials used as ureteral splints. Surg Gynec Obstet 1962; 114: 47–51
22. Abdel-Hakim A, Bernstein J, Teijeira J, Elhilali MM. Urethral stricture after cardiovascular surgery. A retrospective and a prospective study. J Urol 1983; 130: 1100–2
23. Ruutu M, Alfthan O, Heikkinen L et al. Unexpected urethral strictures after short-term catheterization in open-heart surgery. Scand J Urol Nephrol 1984; 18: 9–12
24. Dinneen MD, Wetter LA, May ARL. Urethral strictures and aortic surgery. Suprapubic rather than urethral catheters. Eur J Vasc Surg 1990; 4: 535–8
25. Ruutu M, Alfthan O, Talja M, Andersson LC. Cytotoxicity of latex urinary catheters. Br J Urol 1985; 57: 82–7
26. Abdel-Hakim A, Hassouna M, Teijeira J, Elhilali R. Role of urethral ischemia in the development of urethral strictures after cardiovascular surgery: a preliminary report. J Urol 1985; 131: 1077–9

27. Talja M, Virtanen J, Andersson LC. Toxic catheters and diminished urethral blood circulation in the introduction of urethral strictures. Eur Urol 1986; 12: 340–5

28. Talja M, Anderson LC, Ruutu M, Alfthan O. Toxicity testing of urinary catheters. Br J Urol 1985; 57: 579–84

29. Marx M, Bettman MA, Bridge S et al. The effects of various indwelling ureteral catheter materials on the normal canine ureter. J Urol 1988; 139: 180–5

30. Cormio L, Talja M, Koivusalo A et al. Biocompatibility of various indwelling double-J stents. J Urol. 153: 494–6

31. Mardis HK, Kroeger R. Ureteral stents. Use and complications. Probl Urol 1992; 6: 296–306

32. Mardis HK. Evaluation of polymeric materials for endourologic devices. Emerging importance of hydrogels. Sem Interven Radiol 1987; 4: 36–43

33. Ratner BD, Hoffman AS. Synthetic hydrogels for biomedical applications. In Arrade JD (ed) Hydrogels for medical and related application. ACS Symposium Series, No. 31. Washington, DC, American Chemical Society, 1976; 1

34. Nickel JC, Olson ME, Costerton JW. In vivo coefficient of kinetic friction. Study of urinary catheter biocompatibility. Urology 1987; 29: 501–3

35. Nacey JN, Delahunt B. Toxicity study of first and second generation hydrogel-coated latex urinary catheters. Br J Urol 1991; 67: 314–16

36. Cox AJ. Effect of a hydrogel coating on the surface topography of latex-based urinary catheters: an SEM study. Biomaterials 1987; 8: 500–2

37. Griffith DP, Musher DM, Itin C. Urease. The primary cause of infection-induced urinary stones. Invest Urol 1976; 346–50

38. Cox AJ, Hukins DWL. Morphology of mineral deposits on encrusted urinary catheters investigated by scanning electron microscopy. J Urol 1989; 142: 1347–50

39. Cox AJ, Millington RS, Hukins DWL, Sutton TM. Resistance of catheters coated with a modified hydrogel to encrustation during an in vitro test. Urol Res 1989; 17: 353–6

40. Talja M, Korpela A, Järvi K. Comparison of urethral reaction to full silicone, hydrogen-coated and siliconized latex catheters. Br J Urol 1990; 66: 652–7

41. Keane PF, Bonner MC, Johnston SR et al. Characterization of biofilm and encrustation on ureteric stents in vivo. Br J Urol 1994; 73: 687–91

42. Holmes SAV, Cheng C, Whitfield HN. The development of synthetic polymers that resist encrustation on exposure to urine. Br J Urol 1992; 69: 651–5

43. Zobell CE. The effect of solid surfaces on bacterial activity. J Bacteriol 1943; 46: 39–56

44. Costerton JW, Cheng KJ, Geesey GG et al. Bacterial biofilms in nature and disease. Ann Rev Microbiol 1987; 41: 435–64

45. Nickel JC, Ruseska I, Costerton JW. Tobramycin resistance of cells of Pseudomonas aeruginosa growing as a biofilm on urinary catheter material. Antimicrob Agents Chemother 1985; 27: 619–24

46. Reid G, Denstedt JD, Kang YS et al. Microbial adhesion and biolfilm formation on ureteral stents in vitro and in vivo. J Urol 1992; 148: 1592–4

47. ISO 10993-1: 1992. Biological evaluation of medical devices. Part 1: Evaluation and testing

48. British Standards Institution: Urological catheters, BS 1695: Part 1: 1990

49. United States Pharmacopoeia, 20th edn. United States Pharmacopeial Contention Inc., Rockville MD, 1980

50. Nacey JN, Horsfall DJ, Delahunt B, Marshall VR. The assessment of urinary catheter toxicity using cell cultures: validation by comparison with an animal model. J Urol 1986; 136: 706–9

51. Graham DT, Mark GE, Pomeroy AR. In vivo validation of a cell culture test for biocompatibility testing of urinary catheters. J Biomed Mat Res 1984; 18: 1125–35

52. Ruutu M, Talja M, Andersson LC, Alfthan OS. Biocompatibility of urinary catheters. Scand J Urol Nephrol 1991; 138: 235–8

Alloplastic ureteric replacements and ureteric stents: history, surgical procedures, indications and results

5

L. Cormio   M. Ruutu

Introduction

The existence of a conduit taking down to the bladder the 'moisture' extracted by the kidneys was postulated by Hippocrates, in the fourth century BC. The first detailed anatomical and functional description of the ureter was given by Claudius Galen in the second century AD.[1]

Alloplastic ureteric replacements

Although the ureter has been known for such a long time, there are no descriptions of ureteric replacement operations in the literature before the last decade of the nineteenth century. This is probably due to the fact that the ureter seemed to be an unremarkable conduit between the kidneys and the bladder but mainly because primary diseases of the ureter were quite uncommon. As a matter of fact, the era of ureteric replacement operations started at the end of the nineteenth century due to the need for repairing iatrogenic ureteric injuries following major surgical procedures, such as radical hysterectomy.[2]

Boari was the first to perform an alloplastic replacement of the ureter using a *glass tube* as a conduit between the kidney and bladder in a dog.[3] The experiment was unsuccessful, the dog dying of peritonitis due to urine leakage into the peritoneal cavity. However, this report set into motion the imagination of investigators.

In 1942, Lord and Eckel[4] implanted straight and funnel-shaped *vitallium tubes* into the ureters and renal pelvises of 12 dogs. After 9 months, there was no encrustation nor stone formation. Histologically, only a mild submucosal hyperplasia could be seen at the site where the tip of the funnel-shaped prosthesis was lying. The authors concluded that vitallium tubes could be used in humans for repairing difficult ureteropelvic strictures (funnel-shaped prosthesis) or ureteric injuries (straight prosthesis).

In 1947, Lubash reported his experience with tantalum tubes in the reimplantation of the ureter into the sigmoid colon.[5] The tube was 1-inch long and presented a quarter of an inch long flange on either ends. Both flanges, each representing a small hole to allow the passage of a suture, were

"

sutured to the ureteric stump before its reimplantation into the sigmoid colon. This technique was used in seven dogs, bilaterally in three and unilaterally in four. All four dogs with unilateral reimplantation survived, while two of the three dogs with bilateral reimplantation died because of acute pyelonephritis. However, at autopsy there was no sign of peritonitis nor of anastomotic urine leakage.

Polyethylene tubes were used for the first time in 1949 by Herdman.[6] After having implanted these tubes in the ureters of 15 rabbits, he observed rapid encrustation and blockade, leading to severe hydro-nephrotic changes. A few years later, Tulloch implanted polyethylene tubes in a patient with bilateral ureteric obstruction following hysterectomy.[7] Using a two-stage retroperitoneal approach, he freed the ureter from the ties, incised the stricture and inserted a polyethylene tube into the ureteric lumen with the distal end curled up into the bladder. The tube was removed 9 days later cystoscopically. Both ureteric injuries recovered well. Polyethylene tubes have been subsequently tested in experimental animals by Scher and co-workers.[8] They replaced part of the ureter with a polyethylene tube in four dogs, in one unilaterally and in three bilaterally. Nine months after surgery the tubes were found to be patent and covered by healthy connective tissue. In contrast, using the same material, Hardin[9] observed hydronephrosis due to abolished normal ureteric peristalsis in all the six dogs he had operated on. Moreover, none of the animals survived as long as 6 months.

In 1959, Ulm and Lo published their experience with a double-flanged *polyvinyl tube* in the replacement of dog ureters.[10] The tube was withdrawn into the collecting system through the renal parenchyma using a flexible probe, and the proximal flange fixed to the pelvis. Then the distal part of the tube was withdrawn into the bladder and fixed to the bladder wall. Only three of the 10 dogs they operated on survived longer than one year. They pointed out that the urothelium was not growing along the polyvinyl tube, that encrustation was a major problem with this material, but that flanges represented a valid tool against migration.

One year later, Ulm and Kraus reported their experience with a double-flanged *Teflon tube* in the replacement of dog ureters with the above-mentioned technique.[11] Five of the 10 dogs they operated on survived longer than one year. There was no migration nor encrustation but the tube was found to be 'too rigid for a perfect prosthesis'. Similarly, Warren and co-workers[12] performed partial replacement of the ureter in seven dogs using Teflon grafts with a special Teflon nipple at both ends. The operation failed in all but two dogs due to marked hydronephrosis proximal to the graft, and the authors concluded that Teflon was not a suitable ureteric substitute in their hands.

In 1962, Kocvara and Zak published their study on ureteric substitution with Teflon and *Dacron tubes*.[13] They found that Dacron prostheses with a porous network were not suitable for ureteric substitution due to the penetration of connective tissue and consequent occlusion of the lumen. Conversely, Teflon prostheses healed well without tissue reaction or encrustation.

Silicone rubber prostheses were used for the first time by Blum and co-workers in dogs.[14] All but the distal part of the prosthesis was covered by ivalon. The nude silicon rubber tip was inserted into the bladder extravescally. The ivalon covering was sutured to the outer wall of the bladder and to the ureter. Ten of the 13 prostheses they implanted functioned satisfactorily, while the failures were due to stricture of the ureteroprosthesis anastomosis in two cases and stricture of the vesico-prosthesis anastomosis in one. None of the prostheses presented encrustation. In 1973, Stern and co-workers[15] introduced a silicone rubber prosthesis (Scurasil) with polyethylene glycol terephthalate (Rhodergon) velour cuffs at both ends and a unidirectional valve at the vesical end. Results with this technique have not been universally satisfactory. Of the 17 ureteric replacements performed by Stern and co-workers, 11 failed because the stiff prosthesis acted as a piston in the bladder and renal pelvis, leading to hydronephrosis. Griffith and co-workers[16] reported disappointing results with Dacron-backed silicone rubber tubes, as seven of the 13 prostheses they implanted became completely obstructed due to mucosal plugs in four cases and to angulation in three. Conversely, Djurhuus and co-workers[17] reported good results with this prosthesis. In the five pigs they operated on, the prosthesis did not cause either encrustation, obstruction or hydronephrosis. The only reported complication was late dislodgement. Similarly, Dufour and Blondel[18] and Schulman and co-workers[19] have reported good results in both unilateral and bilateral ureteric replacement in humans. In order to avoid the piston effect of a stiff prosthesis in the bladder and renal pelvis, Schreiber and co-workers[20] developed a prosthesis made of a flexible steel spiral coated with silicone rubber and with Dacron velour cuffs at both ends. None of the 20 pigs they operated on developed hydronephrosis or any other complications, and the authors concluded that this modified prosthesis was well suitable for use in humans.

Promising results have been reported with the use of *polytetrafluoroethy-lene (Gore-tex) tubes* in the replacement of the ureter. In their preliminary report, Dreikorn and co-workers[21] obtained good long-term results in 15 of the 16 ureteric replacements they performed in dogs. In Varady and co-workers experience,[22] however, Gore-tex was well tolerated only when used to bridge gaps between segments of the ureter, while infection and migration occurred when Gore-tex was anastomosed to the bladder.

To avoid the drawback of hydronephrosis, some authors have advocated the use of *'self pumping' ureteric prostheses*. Leandri and co-workers[23] used a silicone rubber prosthesis with an angulation over an antireflux valve and with Rhodergon cuffs at both ends in five patients with satisfactory results. The angulation of the prosthesis allowed variations in length with consequent volume changes which induced suction of urine from the upper part and pumping to the lower part. This flow direction was imposed by the anti-reflux valve. Graw and Bahl[24] have subsequently developed an artificial ureter consisting of two pumping chambers with elastic walls. According to the rhythm of respiration, the two chambers are pressurized via a pneumatic switcher from an intra-abdominal pump. When chamber 1 fills with urine from the renal pelvis, chamber 2 is emptied using breath pressure. When chamber 2 is completely emptied, the pneumatic switcher switches to chamber 1 and empties it during breath. We have not found any reported experience in vivo with this artificial ureter.

Present research in the field of alloplastic ureteric replacement, however, is oriented towards the development of biodegradable scaffolds to be used as templates for spontaneous regeneration of the uroepithelium. Tachibana and co-workers[25] have advocated the use of *collagen sponge tube grafts* for segmental ureteric replacement. They implanted sponge tube grafts in eight dogs, in two without a ureteric stent and in six with a ureteric stent. Leakage and hydronephrosis occurred in the two dogs with the unstented grafts, while the postoperative course was uneventful in the six dogs with stented grafts. Histological examination revealed that the sponge was covered by 5–7 cell layers of uroepithelium and infiltrated by fibroblasts. However, no muscle regeneration could be seen. Atala and co-workers[26] seeded autologous urothelial cells in vitro onto nonwoven meshes of polyglycolic acid polymers and subsequently implanted in vivo the cell–polymer scaffolds. After one month, polymer degradation was evident and the urothelial cells had lined the polymer in continuous layers of 1–3 cell thickness. They concluded that autologous urothelium, reconfigured on a synthetic substrate, may be used in the reconstruction of ureter, bladder and urethra.

Recently, palliative alloplastic replacement of the ureter has been accomplished, in patients with advanced pelvic malignancies causing bilateral ureteric obstruction, by subcutaneous placements of specially designed double-J stents (*subcutaneous nephrovesical diversion*). The upper J is inserted in the renal pelvis percutaneously. Then it is passed subcutaneously through a 2-cm skin incision, and advanced subcutaneously using a Redon stylet.[27] Finally, the lower J is inserted into the bladder using a pre-split trocar. The main complication of this procedure is stent obstruction; in one series[27] it occurred in one out of eight cases, in another[28] in four out of 21 cases. A summary of alloplastic ureteric replacement efforts is given in Table 5.1.

Year	Author	Animal/human	Alloplastic material
1893	Boari [3]	Dog	Glass
1942	Lord and Eckel [4]	Dog	Vitallium
1947	Lubash [5]	Dog	Tantalum
1949	Herdman [6]	Rabbit	Polyethylene
1952	Tulloch [7]	Human	Polyethylene
1954	Hardin [9]	Dog	Polyethylene
1955	Scher et al. [8]	Dog	Polyethylene
1959	Ulm and Lo [10]	Dog	Polyvinyl
1960	Ulm and Krauss [11]	Dog	Teflon
1962	Kocvara and Zak [13]	Dog	Dacron
1963	Warren et al. [12]	Dog	Teflon
1963	Blum et al. [14]	Dog	Silicone covered by ivalon
1973	Stern et al. [15]	Human	Silicone with Rhodergon[R] cuffs
1973	Griffith et al. [16]	Human	Dacron-backed silicone
1974	Djurhuus et al. [17]	Pig	Silicone with Rhodergon[R] cuffs
1975	Dufour and Blondel [18]	Human	Silicone with Rhodergon[R] cuffs
1976	Schulman et al. [19]	Human	Silicone with Rhodergon[R] cuffs
1978	Dreikorn et al. [21]	Dog	Gore-tex[R]
1979	Schreiber et al. [20]	Pig	Silicone-coated steel with Dacron cuffs
1981	Leandri et al. [23]	Human	Angulated silicone with Rhodergon[R] cuffs
1982	Varady et al. [22]	Dog	Gore-tex[R]
1985	Tachibana et al. [25]	Dog	Collagen sponge
1986	Graw and Bahl [24]	In vitro	Artificial self-pumping ureter
1992	Atala et al. [26]	Rat	Urothelial cells on biogradable polymers

Table 5.1. Historical attempts of alloplastic ureteric replacement

Ureteric stents

Ureteric stents were initially used during open surgery, to facilitate upper urinary-tract drainage and to promote ureteric healing. Following the report by Zimskind and co-workers[29] on the clinical use of long-term indwelling silicone stents introduced cystoscopically, much effort has been directed towards development and refinement of internal ureteric stents.

Those stents migrated easily as they had no proximal or distal feature to hold them in place.

To reduce migration, Gibbons and co-workers[30] described a silicone stent with multiple barbs along its shaft and a distal flange. The barbs significantly increased the outer diameter in comparison with the inner one, making proper placement difficult and decreasing the urinary flow rate.[31] Moreover, the distal flange was not capable of preventing migration of the stent towards the urethra.

To prevent both antegrade (towards urethra) and retrograde (towards renal pelvis) migration, the proximal and distal ends of a silicone tube were curved in the shape of a J. Such tips were flexible and could be straightened for stent insertion by an internal guidewire, and returned to the J shape by removing the wire.[32,33] In further development, various forms of hook shape, 'pig-tail' and multicoil constructions have been designed.

Double-J stents have been originally designed to be introduced cysto-scopically. However, these stents can be introduced also percutaneously[34] and even using endoluminal ultrasound.[35]

Indications and results of ureteric stenting

Urolithiasis

This is probably the most common indication for ureteric stenting. Ureteric stenting has been used to manipulate mid or upper ureteric stones into the renal pelvis and to treat them with extracorporeal shock wave lithotripsy (ESWL), with a significantly higher stone-free success rate.[36] Routine ureteric stenting before ESWL treatment of large renal stones has been advocated to prevent the 'steinstrasse' complication.[37,38] Ureteric stenting can also be used to relieve acute ureteric obstruction due to an encased ureteric stone until definitive treatment is performed.[31] Similarly, it can be used to relieve acute ureteric obstruction due to urolithiasis in pregnancy, and to defer definitive treatment in the postpartum period.[39]

Ureteric injuries

Andriole and co-workers[40] first reported a 50% success rate in the management of ureteric fistulas with an indwelling double-J stent. Chang and co-workers[41] reported successful resolution of 10 out of the 12 ureteric fistulas, and of 12 out of the 19 ureteric strictures they treated with percutaneous antegrade ureteric stenting with a double-J catheter. Turner and co-workers[42] have reported good results in 9 of the 10 ureteric fistulas following gynaecological surgery they had treated with an indwelling double-J stent. Similarly, Toporoff and co-workers[43] have reported good results in 5 of the 6 delayed-presenting ureteric injuries secondary to penetrating trauma they had treated with percutaneous antegrade ureteric stenting. In our hands,[44] an attempt to perform ureteric stenting was successful in 16 out of 30 ureteric injuries. However, all injuries treated endourologically healed well. In our experience, ureteric stenting proved to be a valid treatment for recent strictures, less than 2 cm in length, and for small fistulas in which the continuity of the ureteric wall is still partially preserved. Despite the risk of failure, especially following late treatment, it proved to be a safe and effective procedure that is well accepted by the patient and that avoids the need for open surgery and its possible complications. Ureteric stenting has been advocated also for early ureteric obstruction following renal transplantation.[45]

Extrinsic ureteric obstruction

Ureteric stenting has been widely used in the management of ureteric obstruction due to pelvic malignancies or retroperitoneal fibrosis. Andriole and co-workers[40] reported that all 36 patients with advanced pelvic malignancies they had treated with ureteric stenting were hospitalized for less than 4 days and none of them died of uraemia. Similarly, Hoe and co-workers[46] have reported good results in 68% of the uraemic patients with advanced pelvic malignancies they had treated with ureteric stenting.

Urinary drainage following endoscopic ureteric surgery

Ureteric stenting has become a complementary tool to ureteroscopic procedures to prevent either post-ureteroscopic ureteric oedema, or scarring of small mucosal lesions. Kramolowsky and co-workers[47] have reported successful results in 9 (64%) of the 14 ureteric strictures they had treated with endoscopic balloon dilatation and subsequent ureteric stenting. Similarly, Netto and co-workers[48] have reported a 57% success rate for the ureteric strictures they initially had treated with balloon dilation and subsequent ureteric stenting. Ureteric stenting has been reported to be useful also in connection with endopyelotomy and endoureterotomy for benign strictures.[49,51]

Urinary drainage following open ureteric surgery

Although ureteric stenting is widely used to promote ureteric healing after end-to-end ureterostomy, pyeloplasty and uretero-enteral diversions, the dilemma of 'to stent or not to stent' is far from being solved.

Extensive studies were conducted at the end of the 1950s to determine whether or not ureteric stenting promotes ureteric healing. McDonald and Calams[52] have pointed out that ureteric healing is the same whether a stent is present or not. Conversely, Oppenheimer and Hinman[53] have proved that ureteric stents promote ureteric healing by providing a scaffold for epithelialization and by avoiding early flow of urine through the defect.

In a valuable review of the pathophysiology of ureteric healing and ureteric stenting, Lee and Smith[54] have recently concluded that the use of stents during open ureteric surgery is a matter of surgical judgement, and that ureteric stenting is mandatory only when long suture lines are present or when there is a risk of distal ureteric obstruction.

Prevention of ureteric injuries during open surgery

Preoperative ureteric stenting has been recommended in the past to prevent ureteric injuries due to gynaecological procedures[55] as well as those due to general surgical procedures.[56] The experience gained over the years has shown that preoperative catheterization is not effective in preventing the trauma[57] and could even provoke it.[58,59] Recently, the use of transilluminating ureteric stents has been advocated for preventing ureteric injuries during gynaecological procedures.[60]

Complications of ureteric stenting

The usage of double-J ureteric stents is not free from problems, several complications having been reported in the literature.

Symptoms

Symptoms may arise and be troublesome in patients with indwelling ureteric stents.[61] Loin pain, characteristically sharp during voiding, may occur in as much as 50% of the patients with indwelling stents because of vesico-ureteric reflux and consequent increase in intrapelvic pressure. Also dysuria, nocturia, frequency and lower abdominal pain in the absence of urinary infection may occur in as much as 50% of the patients with indwelling stents due to the irritative effect exerted by the foreign material. In most cases, stent removal leads to resolution of the symptoms.

The incidence of symptoms does not seem to be related to the stent material,[62] but to the indwelling time; the longer the time, the higher the related morbidity.[63]

Migration

Migration in either direction may occur despite the J shape of the stent and can be problematic. Stents with a full coil rarely migrate, unlike those with the J shape. The composition of the stent may also affect migration: polyurethane stents have the best memory, thus the least tendency to migrate, whereas silicone stents have the least memory and consequently the highest tendency to migrate.[31]

Encrustation and breakage

Encrustation and consequent breakage are also well-known complications. From the moment a stent is placed in the urinary milieu, mucoproteins attach to its surface. Following encrustation will depend on the degree of crystalloid supersaturation in the urine.[64] Ramsay and co-workers[65] proved that the barium or bismuth used to make the stent radiopaque leached from the polymer and was incorporated into the encrustation. Holmes and co-workers[66] have recently confirmed that encrustation depends on the chemical composition of the stent material and have proved that the incorporation of fluorine-containing components confers significant resistance to the formation of encrustation.

Infection

The relationship between indwelling stents and the development of urinary-tract infection is unclear. In a recent study,[67] the incidence of urinary infection in patients with indwelling stents was 7.5%, based upon urine culture. However, the patients were given antibiotic coverage. In another study,[68] in which the patients had no antibiotic coverage, the incidence of urinary infection was 27%. Moreover, as much as 90% of the stents were found to be colonized by adherent uropathogens. The ability of uropathogens to adhere to the uroepithelium or to the surface of prosthetic devices is recognized as an important mechanism in the initiation and pathogenesis of urinary infection.[69] The correlation between biofilm formation and infection, however, does not always apply in vivo as bacterial biofilms have been found on intrauterine devices and peritoneal catheters without infection arising.[70] The development of infection-resistant polymers, currently under investigation, would be desirable to prevent such complications.

Hydrodynamic changes in the upper urinary tract

Hydrodynamic changes in the upper urinary tract are known to occur in patients with indwelling stents. Ramsay and co-workers[71] found in vivo that most of the urinary flow from the renal pelvis to the bladder occurred by bolus propagation around the ureteric stent, urine only flowing through the lumen when an obstruction prevented the forward movement of the ureteric peristaltic waves. Payne and Ramsay[72] proved that acute ureteric stenting caused a great rise in intrapelvic pressure, the magnitude of which depended on the size of the stent. Intrapelvic pressure returned to normal values after three weeks' intubation. This phenomenon was attributed to a mild ureteric dilatation following intubation. They concluded that double-J stents provided only a suboptimal renal drainage. Mosli and associates[73] have questioned the safety of double-J stents as they found vesico-ureteric reflux and reduction in ureteric peristaltic activity in most (80%) of their patients with stents.

If spontaneous adaptation to these hydrodynamic changes and restoration of the baseline hydrodynamic situation does not occur within three weeks, ureteric stenting may have deleterious effects on renal function.

Effects on the uroepithelium

Ramsay and co-workers[71] first pointed out that porcine ureters responded to three weeks' intubation with polyurethane stents with a generalized thickening of the wall, hyperplasia and mucous metaplasia of the epithelium. More recently, Marx and co-workers[74] have studied the effects of various indwelling double-J stent materials on the normal canine ureter. They found that after six weeks of intubation, epithelial ulceration was prominent in ureters stented with pure polyurethane and infrequent in ureters stented with silicone, C-Flex™ (polysiloxane) or Silitek™ (a proprietary, silicone-containing elastomer), while oedema was more marked in ureters stented with Silitek™ than in ureters stented with other materials. They concluded that silicone and C-Flex™ stents were more suitable for ureteric stenting than the other tested materials. Damage to the uroepithelium may be responsible for the irritative symptoms observed in patients with indwelling stents.

Conclusions

Despite some enthusiastic reports, alloplastic ureteric replacement has never definitely come into clinical use because of the large number of drawbacks associated with their use, lack of knowledge about their biocompatibility in the long term and, mainly, the availability of internal ureteric stents. Ureteric stents have become a fundamental tool of the urological armamentarium. They can be used alternatively to nephrostomy tubes in selected cases of ureteric obstruction, fistula, trauma or stone. In the absence of ureteric pathology, however, the dilemma of 'to stent or not to stent' is far from being solved. Ureteric wall thickening and epithelial changes, as well as hydrodynamic conditions caused by indwelling stents, such as ureteric dilatation, increased renal pelvic pressure, vesico-ureteric reflux and extraluminal urine flow, support the non-stenting policy whenever this is not strictly necessary. It is possible that stents cause more harm than benefit, but because the results with their routine use are usually good, it is difficult to prove such a conclusion.

References

1. Hovnanian AP. Ureteral replacements. Surg Gynecol Obstet 1972; 135: 801–10
2. Wertheim F. Zur Frage der Radikaloperation bei Uteruskrebs. Arch Gynaecol 1900; 61: 627–31
3. Boari A. Cited by Hovnanian AP. Ureteral replacements. Surg Gynecol Obstet 1972; 135: 801–10
4. Lord JW, Eckel JH. The use of vitallium tubes in the urinary tract of dogs. J Urol 1942; 48: 412–20

5. Lubash S. Experience with tantalum tubes in the reimplantation of the ureters into the sigmoids in dogs and humans. J Urol 1947; 57: 1010–27

6. Herdman JP. Polyethylene tubing in the experimental surgery of the ureter. Br J Surg 1949; 37: 105–6

7. Tullock WS. Restoration of continuity of the ureter by means of a polyethylene tubing. Br J Urol 1952; 24: 42–5

8. Scher AM, Erikson RV, Scher M. Polyethylene as partial ureteral prosthesis in dogs. J Urol 1955; 73: 987–9

9. Hardin CA. Experimental repair of the ureters by polyethylene tubing and ureteral and vessel grafts. Arch Surg 1954; 68: 57–61

10. Ulm AH, Lo MC. Total bilateral polyvinyl ureteral substitutes in the dog. Surgery 1959; 45: 313–20

11. Ulm AH and Kraus L. Total unilateral Teflon ureteral substitutes in the dog. J Urol 1960; 83: 575–82

12. Warren JW Jr, Coomer T, Fransen H. The use of Teflon for replacementt of ureters. II. J Urol 1963; 89: 164–6

13. Kocvara S and Zak F. Ureteral susbtitution with Dacron and Teflon prostheses. J Urol 1962; 88: 365–76

14. Blum J, Skemp C, Reiser M. Silicone rubber ureteral prosthesis. J Urol 1963; 90: 276–80

15. Stern A, Apoli A, Thony H et al. A silicone polyester prosthesis for ureteral replacement. Trans Am Soc Artif Int Organs 1973; 19: 370–5

16. Griffith DP, Moseley WG, Beach PD. Experimental studies in ureteral substitution. Invest Urol 1973; 11: 239–43

17. Djurhuus JC, Gyrd-Hansen N, Nerstrom B, Svenson O. Total replacement of ureter by a Scurasil prosthesis in pig. Br J Urol 1974; 46: 415–24

18. Dufour B, Blondel P. The prosthetic replacement of the ureter. Experimental and clinical results. Eur Urol 1975; 1: 134–9

19. Schulman CC, Vanderdris M, Vanlanduyt P, Abramow M. Total replacement of both ureters by prostheses. Eur Urol 1976; 2: 89–91

20. Schreiber B, Homann W, Mlynek M, Mellin P. Ureteral replacement with a new prosthesis. Trans Am Soc Artif Int Organs 1979; 25: 61–3

21. Dreikorn K, Löbelenz J, Horsch R, Röhl L. Alloplastic replacement of the canine ureter by expanded polytetrafluoroethylene (Gore-tex[R]) grafts. Eur Urol 1978; 4: 379–81

22. Varady S, Friedman E, Yap WT et al. Ureteral replacement with a new synthetic material: Gore-tex. J Urol 1982; 128: 171–5

23. Leandri J, Abbou C, Rey P. Human application of a self-pumping ureteral prosthesis. Trans Am Soc Artif Int Organs 1981; 27: 336–40

24. Graw M, Bahl HU. An active artificial ureter with autonomous energy supply. Eur Urol 1986; 41: 9–15

25. Tachibana M, Nagamatsu GR, Addonizio JC. Ureteral replacement using collagen sponge tube grafts. J Urol 1985; 133: 866–9

26. Atala A, Vacanti JP, Peters CA et al. Formation of urothelial structures in vivo from dissociated cells attached to biodegradable polymer scaffolds in vitro. J Urol 1992; 148: 658–62

27. Ahmadzadeh M. Clinical experience with subcutaneous urinary diversion: new approach using a double pigtail stent. Br J Urol 1991; 67: 596–9

28. Di Lelio A. Circumvallate nephro-cystostomy. Arch Ital Urol Nefrol Androl 1992; 64(suppl 2): 45–9

29. Zimskind PD, Fetter TR, Wilkerson JL. Clinical use of long-term indwelling silicone rubber ureteral splints inserted cystoscopically. J Urol 1967; 97: 840–3

30. Gibbons RP, Correa RJ Jr, Cummings KB, Mason JT. Experience with indwelling ureteral stent catheters. J Urol 1976; 115: 22–6

31. Saltzman B. Ureteral stents. Indications, variations and complications. Urol Clin N Am 1988; 15: 481–91

32. Finney RP. Experience with new double-J ureteral catheter stent. J Urol 1978; 120: 678–81

33. Hepperlen TW, Mardis HK, Kammendel H. Self-retained internal ureteral stents: a new approach. J Urol 1978; 119: 731–4

34. Kahn RI. Percutaneous antegrade indwelling silicone stent. Urology 1986; 27: 467–9

35. Wolf MC, Hollander JB, Salisz JA, Kearney DJ. A new technique for ureteral stent placement during pregnancy using endoluminal ultrasound. Surg Gynecol Obstet 1992; 175: 575–6

36. Riehle RA, Naslond EN. Treatment of calculi in the upper ureter with extracorporeal shock wave lithotripsy. Surg Gynecol Obstet 1987; 164: 1–8

37. Riehle RA. Selective use of ureteral stents before extracorporeal shock wave lithotripsy. Urol Clin N Am 1988; 15: 499–506

38. Shabsigh R, Gleeson MJ, Griffith DP. The benefits of stenting on more-or-less routine basis prior to extracorporeal shock wave lithotripsy. Urol Clin N Am 1988; 15: 493–7

39. Loughlin KR, Bailey JR. Internal ureteral stents for conservative management of ureteral calculi during pregnancy. New Engl J Med 1986; 315: 1647–9

40. Andriole GL, Bettmann MA, Garnick MB, Richie JP. Indwelling double-J ureteral stents for temporary and permanent urinary drainage: experience with 87 patients. J Urol 1984; 131: 239–41

41. Chang R, Marshall FF, Mitchell S. Percutaneous management of benign ureteral strictures and fistulas. J Urol 1987; 137: 1126–31

42. Turner WH, Cranston DW, Davies AH et al. Double-J stents in the treatment of gynaecological injury to the ureter. J R Soc Med 1990; 83: 623–4

43. Toporoff B, Sclafani S, Scalea T et al. Percutaneous antegrade ureteral stenting as an adjunct for treatment of complicated ureteral injuries. J Trauma 1992; 32: 534–8

44. Cormio L, Battaglia M, Traficante A, Selvaggi FP. Endourological treatment of ureteric injuries. Br J Urol 1993; 72: 165–7

45. Berger RE, Ansel JS, Tremann JA et al. The use of self-retained ureteral stents in the management of urologic complications in renal transplant recipients. J Urol 1980; 124: 781–2

46. Hoe JWM, Tung KH, Tan EC. Re-evaluation of indications for percutaneous nephrostomy and interventional uro-radiological procedures in pelvic malignancy. Br J Urol 1993; 71: 469–72

47. Kramolowsky EV, Tucker RD, Nelson CMK. Management of benign ureteral strictures: open surgical repair or endoscopic dilation? J Urol 1989; 141: 285–6

48. Netto NR Jr, Ferreira U, Lemos GC, Claro JFA. Endourological management of ureteral strictures. J Urol 1990; 144: 631–4

49. Schneider AW, Busch R, Otto U, Klosterhalfen H. Endourological management of 41 stenosis in the upper urinary tract using the cold knife technique. J Urol 1989; part 2, 141: 208A, abstract 155

50. Franco I, Eshghi M, Schwalb D, Addonizio JC. Cold knife endoureterotomy of 28 ureteral strictures. J Urol 1989; part 2, 141: 208A, abstract 158.

51. Meretyk S, Albala DM, Clayman RV et al. Endoureterotomy for treatment of ureteral strictures. J Urol 1992; 147: 1502–6

52. McDonald JH, Calams JA. Experimental ureteral stricture: ureteral regrowth following ureterotomy with or without intubation. J Urol 1960; 84: 52–9

53. Oppenheimer R, Hinman F Jr. The effect of urinary flow upon ureteral regeneration in the absence of splint. Surg Gynecol Obstet 1956; 103: 416–22

54. Lee CK, Smith AD. Role of stents in open ureteral surgery. J Endourol 1993; 7: 141–4

55. Valk WL, Foret JD. The problem of vesico-vaginal and uretero-vaginal fistulas. Med Clin N Am 1959; 43: 1769–75

56. Remington JH. Prevention of ureteral injury in surgery of the pelvic colon. Dis Colon Rectum 1959; 2: 340–9

57. Leff EI, Groff W, Rubin RJ et al. Use of ureteral catheters in colonic and rectal surgery. Dis Colon Rectum 1982; 25: 457–60

58. Selvaggi FP, Battaglia M, Traficante A et al. Obstetric and gynecological lesions of the ureter: experience with 88 injuries. Int Urogynecol J 1991; 2: 81–4

59. Sheikh FA, Khubchandani IT. Prophylactic ureteric catheters in colon surgery – how safe are they? Report of three cases. Dis Colon Rectum 1990; 33: 508–10

60. Phipps JH, Tyrrell NJ. Transilluminating ureteric stents for preventing operative ureteric damage. Br J Obstet Gynaecol 1992; 99: 81

61. Pollard SG, Macfarlane R. Symptoms arising from double-J ureteral stents. J Urol 1988; 139: 37–8

62. Pryor JL, Langley MJ, Jenkins AD. Comparison of symptom characteristics of indwelling ureteral catheters. J Urol 1991; 145: 719–22
63. El-faqih SR, Shamsuddin AB, Chakrabarti A et al. Polyurethane internal ureteral stents in treatment of stone patients: morbidity related to indwelling time. J Urol 1991; 146: 1487–91
64. Mardis HK, Kroeger R. Ureteral stents. Use and complications. Probl Urol 1992; 6: 296–306
65. Ramsay JWA, Crocker RP, Ball AJ et al. Urothelial reaction to ureteric intubation. A clinical study. Br J Urol 1987; 60: 504–5
66. Holmes SAV, Cheng C, Whitfield HN. The development of synthetic polymers that resist encrustation on exposure to urine. Br J Urol 1992; 69: 651–5
67. Franco G, De Dominicis C, Dal Formo S et al. The incidence of post-operative urinary tract infection in patients with ureteric stents. Br J Urol 1990; 65: 10–12
68. Reid G, Denstedt JD, Kany YS et al. Microbial adhesion and biofilm formation on ureteral stents in vitro and in vivo. J Urol 1992; 148: 1592–4
69. Costerton JW, Cheng KJ, Geesey GG et al. Bacterial biofilm in nature and disease. Annu Rev Microbiol 1987; 41: 435–64
70. Dasgupta M, Costerton JW. Significance of biofilm-adherent bacterial microcolonies on Tenckhoff catheters of CAPD patients. Blood Purification 1989; 7: 144–55
71. Ramsay JWA, Payne SR, Gosling PT et al. The effects of double J stenting on unobstructed ureters. An experimental and clinical study. Br J Urol 1985; 57: 630–4
72. Payne SR, Ramsay JWA. The effects of double J stents on renal pelvic dynamics in the pig. J Urol 1988; 140: 637–41
73. Mosli HA, Farsi HMA, Fawzi Al-Zimaity M et al. Vesicoureteral reflux in patients with double pigtail stents. J Urol 1991; 146: 966–9
74. Marx M, Bettmann MA, Bridge S et al. The effects of various indwelling ureteral catheter materials on the normal canine ureter. J Urol 1988; 139: 180–5

Urethral stents: history, surgical procedure, indication and results for treating BPH, urethral stricture and neurological voiding dysfunction

6

G. Williams

Introduction

In 1980 Fabian reported the use of a stainless-steel coil as a stent in the prostatic urethra in patients who would otherwise have been treated with a long-term urethral catheter.[1] Implanting such devices into the urinary tract is likely to lead to encrustation and recurrent infection. To reduce the incidence of these complications, modifications of the original stainless-steel spiral have taken place and several new stents introduced. These stents are referred to as temporary stents in that they are not incorporated into the urinary tract and can be removed with relative ease. They have been used both in the treatment of prostatic obstruction and urethral strictures (Table 6.1).

Prostate
- Urospiral
- Intraurethral catheter
- Prostacoil
- Prostacath
- Memocath
- P-spring

Urethra
- Urocoil
- Intraurethral catheter

Table 6.1. Temporary stents/catheters

The findings that stents manufactured of a woven mesh of super-alloy, titanium or nickel/titanium would become covered with normal urothelium when the stent was held against the wall of the urinary tract by the radial force of the device, led to the introduction in 1987 of so-called permanently implanted stents (Table 6.2). These have been used to treat

---

Prostate
- Urolume
- Titan
- Memotherm
- Gianturco
- Ultraflex

Urethra
- Urolume
- Memotherm
- Titan

Sphincter
- Urolume

Table 6.2. Permanently implanted stents

prostatic obstruction, urethral strictures and neurological voiding disorders. Such stents are still undergoing modification and as a result the reported follow-up is often short. Whereas temporary prostatic stents are becoming more permanent, with follow-up of some patients of greater than four years, permanently implanted prostatic stents appear to be becoming more temporary.

In 1988 Milroy reported use of the original Urolume[TM] (American Medical Systems) permanently implanted stent for the treatment of bulbar strictures which had recurred after previous treatments.[2] In 1989, Williams et al. used the same Urolume[TM] stent in patients with prostatic obstruction[3] and in 1990 Shaw et al.[4] used this stent in patients with neurological voiding disorders as a result of spinal injury.

Permanently implanted stents for the treatment of prostatic obstruction

Urolume[TM]

The Urolume[TM] stent is a woven tubular mesh of corrosion-resistant super-alloy wire manufactured to various lengths. Since its first introduction in 1987 for the treatment of urethral strictures, it has as a result of both technical and clinical complications undergone at least two modifications, with the result that the follow-up of the latest commercially available stent is considerably limited. The original indication was for men who were unfit for prostatic surgery. However, it became clear that the insertion of a stent into the prostatic urethra resulted in severe dysuria, frequency and urgency in a significant proportion of the patients studied and though the symptoms resolved in the majority by three months, often with the additional use of anticholinergics, they were a major disadvantage

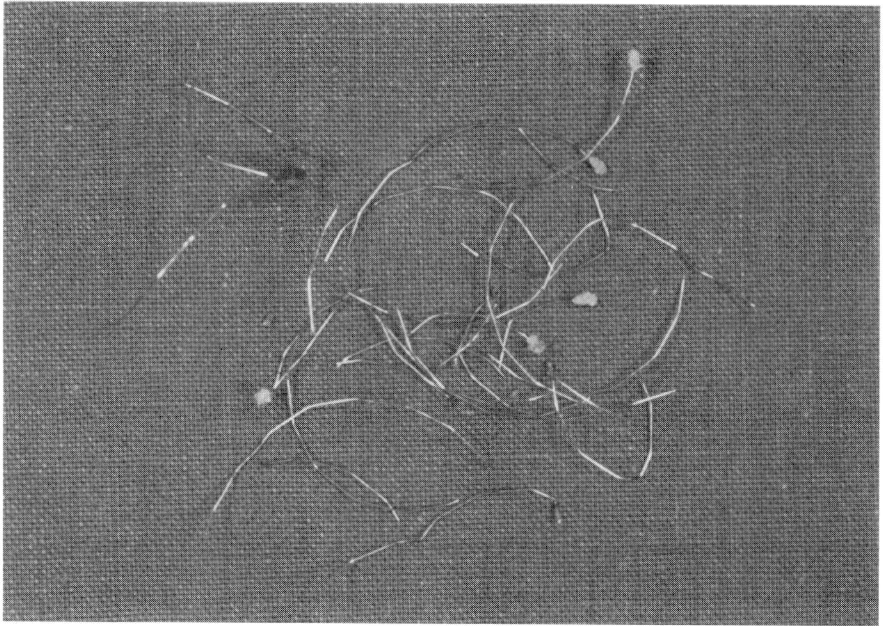

Fig. 6.1. A Urolume^{TM} stent removed piecemeal showing calcification on some of the wires.

to those elderly, unfit men for whom they were supposed to benefit. In addition, should it become necessary, this stent is not easy to remove, particularly when it has become incorporated into the prostatic urethra. Though on occasions it can be dislodged after resection of the lining urothelium and pulled into the sheath of a resectoscope, it is more common to have to break the stent and remove it piecemeal (Fig. 6.1). This is a long and often bloody procedure and may delay the performance of a definitive treatment in a patient already deemed unfit for surgery.

Indications

As the majority of men maintain antegrade ejaculation and potency, the use of the stent might be indicated in a man who is fit for surgery but declines and where preservation of potency and antegrade ejaculation is important.

Contraindications

The presence of a large middle lobe or bladder neck and a large rigid prostate which prevents full stent expansion.

Technique of insertion

Most authors have used prophylactic antibiotics around the time of stent insertion. The original stent delivery system consisted of a small-diameter catheter on which a doubled-over plastic membrane held the stent in a compressed and elongated state. This stent was inserted under radiological or ultrasound guidance. Since 1990 the stent has been inserted on a specially made disposable endoscopic delivery device. Patients are sedated or given light anaesthesia and placed in the lithotomy position. A diagnostic cystourethroscopy is performed and the length of the prostatic urethra measured with the bladder full, using a graduated balloon occlusion catheter placed at the bladder neck. The distance from the bladder neck to the external sphincter is measured. A stent 0.5 cm shorter than this distance is used. The stent is packaged and mounted in the disposable delivery device. It must be ensured that the two safety locks are in the proper position to prevent premature release of the stent. The delivery device is introduced into the prostatic urethra under direct vision using a standard zero-degree telescope and water irrigation. When in position the first safety lock is released and the stent deployed within the urethra by gently squeezing the trigger mechanism which pulls back the covering sheath, allowing the stent to expand. When the covering sheath has been pulled back as far as the second safety lock, the position of the stent is checked by moving the telescope along the full length of the stent. If the position of the stent is not correct the outer covering sheath can be pushed forwards over the device allowing repositioning. The stent should not intrude over the bladder neck as these wires will not become epithelialized and may calcify. Should the patient be unable to void following stent insertion, a suprapubic catheter must be inserted. The insertion of a urethral catheter in this situation is likely to dislodge the stent into the bladder. Some patients can be dealt with as a day case but those who are unfit may need to be in hospital for a number of days until the frequency and urgency resolves to an acceptable level.

Results

Interpretation of the published results is difficult as it is frequently not stated which stent has been used. In addition, many studies have been multicentred. Apart from the inherent difficulties in interpreting the results of multicentre studies, particularly when small numbers were inserted in many centres, a number were performed in the United States and Europe where the cost of invasive follow-up, such as urodynamics or cystoscopy, is borne by the patient. As a result, these investigations are frequently not performed, leading to a possible underreporting of complications or side effects. There is a learning curve with regard to the technique of insertion and removal. This also influences the results.

Study 1[5]

In this study we contributed 46 of the 96 patients using the original stent in patients unfit for surgery. All patients were able to void following stent insertion and at the latest follow-up which ranged from 1 to 60 months the mean peak flow in those able to void a volume of >150 ml was 18 ml/s with a range of 3–36 ml/s. The mean obstructive score was 0.5 with a range of 0–3 and irritative score of 2.6 with a range of 0–11 (Madsen Iversen system). It became clear from this study that the stent should not be inserted with wires projecting over the bladder neck and that on release from its delivery device the stent shortened to a variable degree. As a result, the original stent was modified and used in a second study for men fit for surgery.

Study 2[6,7]

We contributed 44 patients to this study using the new less-shortening stent in men who were fit for surgery. Follow-up is from 12 to 30 months and again all 44 patients were able to void. The mean peak flow at the latest period of follow-up was 16.1 ml/s with a range of 3–35 ml/s, an obstructive score of 1.6 with a range of 0–10 and an irritative score of 2.5 with a range of 0–7. Because of the complications seen with this stent it is not being marketed and a new stent is now being studied as an alternative to the transurethral resection in a randomized study. We are not participating in this study as the long-term effects of this new stent are unknown. Despite this, the stent is being marketed. The complications seen in these two studies are shown in Table 6.3. Irritable symptoms which may include pain, dysuria, frequency, urgency and urge incontinence are almost invariable following stent insertion but are helped by reassurance, anticholinergics and time. In the majority of patients, these irritable symptoms have resolved by three months, but in some they persist and may lead to the patient requesting the stent to be removed. Severe hyperplasia of the urothelium within the stent was a feature of the second study with the less-shortening stent, as was stent migration. Hyperplasia, persistent

Parameter	Study 1	Study 2
n	46	44
Removal	5	15
Migration	2	10
Hyperplasia	2	7
Calcification	7	1
< 50% epithelialization	1	0
Irritability < 3 months	40	32
Irritability > 3 months	12	7
Second procedure stent	0	0
BNI	0	1
TURP	5	14

Table 6.3. Complications of prostate stents (Urolume)
BNI=Bladder neck incision
TURP=Transurethral resection of the prostate

irritable symptoms and migration led to the stent being removed in 15 of the 44 patients. This incidence of stent removal or replacement is similar to that found in larger multicentred European studies. As these stents cost around 1500 US$ the cost-effectiveness of any new stent needs to be closely studied in large single-centre trials prior to marketing.

The Memotherm™ stent (Angiomed)

This stent is made from woven nitinol, a mixture of nickel and titanium, and is dependent on shape memory. When cold, the stent is compressible, distortable and flexible, but when warmed to body temperature it expands to a 42 Fr cylinder. It is available in lengths from 2 to 8 cm and when released from its delivery device, it does not shorten. It is also easy to remove as the stent unravels when the terminal wire is pulled.

Method of insertion

A preliminary cystourethroscopy is performed and the distance from the bladder neck to the external sphincter is measured using a graduated balloon occlusion catheter. The stent is available in a pre-packed sterile disposable endoscopic delivery device (Fig. 6.2). The proximal 1 cm of the stent is gold-plated to aid visualization. Using a zero-degree telescope and irrigation fluid warmed to body temperature, the endoscope is passed and the bladder neck visualized. The safety catch (Fig. 6.2) is removed and the stent expelled from the delivery device by repeatedly squeezing the trigger

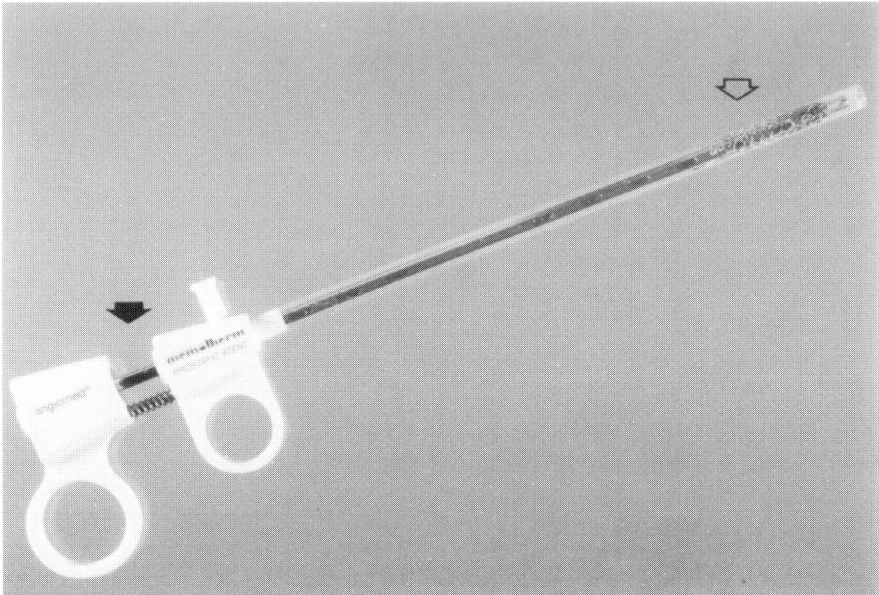

Fig. 6.2. The Memotherm™ delivery device. Black arrow = position of safety catch. Open arrow = proximal gold colouring of the compressed stent on the delivery device.

mechanism. Once the gold colouring is visualized, the position of the stent is checked and the position adjusted. It becomes increasingly difficult to adjust the stent position once more if the stent is deployed. It is not posssible, unlike the Urolume^{TM} stent, to reinsert the Memotherm into the delivery device once it has been deployed. Used with warmed irrigation fluid, the stent immediately expands to 42 Fr. If the patient is unable to void, a suprapubic catheter must be inserted.

Indications

It is unlikely that the original version of the stent will continue to be marketed (see Results). It is expensive but easy to remove.

Contraindications

Bladder-neck hyperplasia, a large middle lobe of the prostate.

Results

Forty-nine stents were inserted into 48 men as an alternative to a transurethral resection. As this was a study of a new stent, there were no exclusions. Follow-up was at 1, 3, 6, and 12 months with flow rates, symptom scores (Madsen Iversen) and cystoscopy at 6 and 12 months. Only 35 patients were able to void following stent insertion, the remainder requiring a suprapubic catheter for up to 11 weeks. Ten stents were removed (Table 6.4). The two patients with incontinence had severe neurological disorders. Obstructive scores at 6 months are shown in Fig. 6.3 and the irritative scores in Fig. 6.4. The subjective benefits seen in the symptom scores were not borne out by the peak urine flow rate at 6 months (Fig. 6.5). Cystoscopy at 6 months in 33 patients showed distal migration in seven, proximal migration in two, hyperplasia in 11, 100%

Stents removed ($n = 10$)

Patient reference number	Time (weeks)	Reason
2	9	Incontinence
4	2	Incontinence
7	4	Irritation
8	11	Irritation
9	11	Failure to void
13	1	Total migration
15	28	Dislodged at cystoscopy
28	1	Total migration
40	1	Incontinence
45	1	Total migration

Table 6.4. Memotherm results (n = 49)

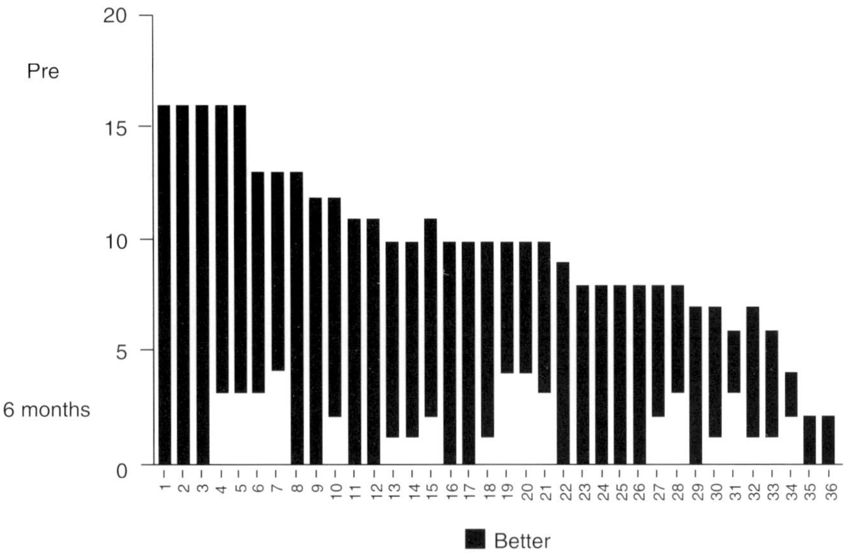

Fig. 6.3. Obstructive scores (Madsen Iversen) at 6 months showing a general improvement (n = 36).

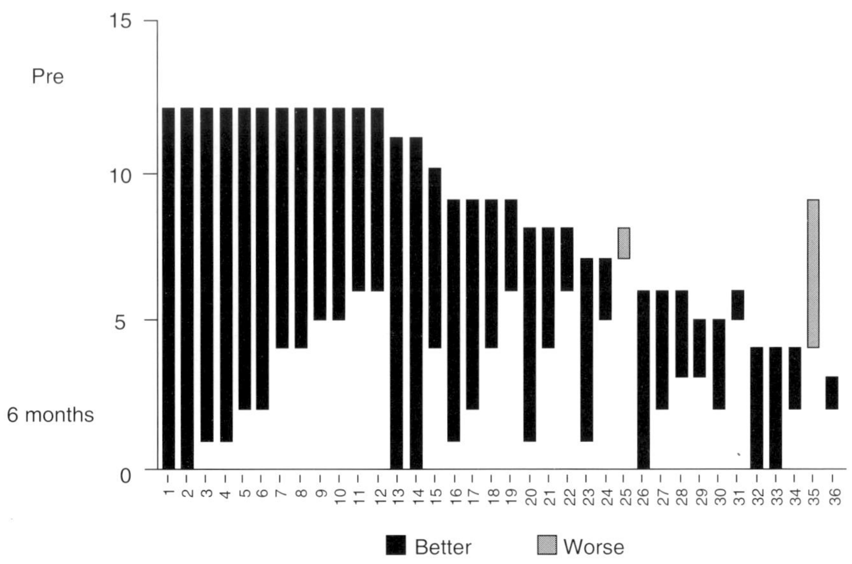

Fig. 6.4. Irritative scores (Madsen Iversen) at 6 months showing an improvement in the majority of patients (n = 36).

epithelialization in five, 75% epithelialization in 17, less than 50% epithelialization in seven and calcification in one.

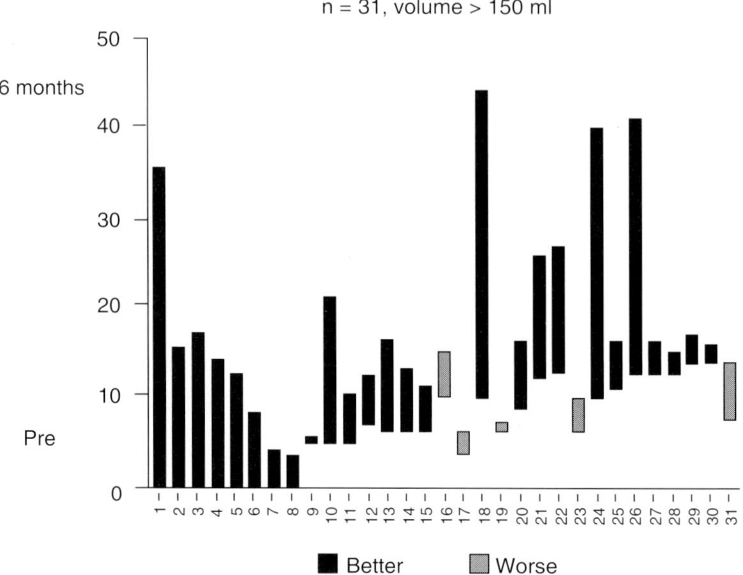

Fig. 6.5. Peak urinary flow (ml/s) at 6 months showing little or no improvement in the majority of patients (n = 31, volume > 150 ml).

This stent, though still marketed, is to undergo significant modification before being subjected to further clinical trials.

The titanium stent

This stent is made of titanium and both the stent and its delivery system continue to undergo further modification. The original stent was manufactured by ASI, California, and was known as the ASI Prostate Dilatation System (PDS). This was a pure titanium mesh stent. It was modified so that the width of the bars of the stent decreased and the fenestrations between the bars made smaller and more numerous. The delivery device was also changed. It is difficult to tell from the published data which stent is being described. In the study by Kaplan et al.[8] 45 patients were treated with the PDS system and 23 with the Titan™ intraprostatic stent. However, the results are combined despite the fact that 17 of the PDS stents had to be removed and none of the Titan™ stents. Urine flow data were available in 25 patients with a stent in situ for greater than one year. Only four patients had a peak urinary flow of more than 15 ml/s. Only mean data for obstructive and irritative scores, flow rate and residual urine are reported. In a longer term UK study of 135 patients with a mean follow-up of 21 months, 95 patients were treated with the original stent and 40 with the newly designed stent; 86% were able to void, but only 10 patients underwent further cystoscopic examination,[9] despite a higher in vitro risk of encrustation.[10] Data from the manufacturers on 207 patients included

170 who were available for follow-up. At 12 months, the average peak urine flow was only 10.9 ml/s suggesting that a significant proportion of these patients were still obstructed probably as a result of hyperplastic urothelium.[11] Though earlier results have suggested that this stent was a satisfactory alternative to prostatectomy in high-risk patients[12,13] this has not been borne out by longer term follow-up and the stent is currently unavailable.

Other permanently implantable prostatic stents have too short a follow-up to warrant further description at this stage. The prostatic urethra is not cylindrical and the bladder neck is not static. Any device inserted into the prostatic urethra will be subjected to the static and dynamic forces of the prostate. A permanently implanted prostatic stent needs to be fixed in position so that it does not migrate. It needs to be in contact with the urothelium so that it becomes incorporated by it and it needs to be able to withstand the compressive forces surrounding it.

The new materials being used for the production of these stents are biocompatible but the diameter of the wires and the distance between them is obviously crucial. Some men undoubtedly do well once the initial irritative symptoms have subsided but the longest follow-up of the original stents is still only five years and most of those patients who were unfit for surgery have died. Second-generation stents are not being marketed (Urolume[TM] and Titan[TM]).

Permanently implanted prostatic stents should still be considered experimental, and should be studied in units where large numbers of patients are available and invasive investigation and follow-up with cystoscopy and urodynamics can be performed. They are expensive and should not be marketed until the results of a cost–benefit analysis is known.

Temporary prostatic stents

These have been available since 1978 and were originally intended as a short-term alternative to the use of an indwelling urethral catheter.[1] The original stent was made of stainless steel and was prone to migration, calcification and recurrent urinary infections. With modifications in design and materials, these so-called temporary stents are being used with increasing frequency to relieve bladder outflow obstruction for four years or more.[14]

Indications

The current indications for temporary stents are as an alternative to a urethral catheter in patients with bladder outflow obstruction who are temporarily or permanently unfit for surgery or who have a short life expectancy. In some countries, for example the UK where there is only one urologist per 170 000 of the population, they are also being used to provide treatment where there is a long waiting list for surgery. Less frequently they are used to assess the probable benefits of surgery in patients with neurological disorders, which may affect voiding, for example Parkinson's disease. If patients remain continent following insertion of a stent, they may either undergo definitive surgery or keep the stent in situ. Temporary stents are considerably less expensive than permanent stents and may be used as an alternative.

Technique of insertion

A preliminary cystourethroscopy should always be performed. Temporary prostatic stents, once inserted, do not permit the passage of an endoscope. The distance between the bladder neck and the external sphincter does not need to be as accurately measured as for a permanently implanted prostatic stent. In all types of temporary stents, the stent is allowed to project into the bladder. Measurement of the prostatic urethral length can be undertaken by ultrasound, a graduated balloon occlusion catheter or a ureteric catheter passed alongside the endoscope. The method of insertion for each of the devices mentioned in Table 6.1 varies: some are simply pushed with an endoscope along the urethra, their position being assessed either with ultrasound or direct vision; others have a special delivery device and reference should be made to the manufacturer's instructions. In most patients the stent can be inserted using topical local anaesthesia. Patients with a known urinary infection should receive a full course of antibiotic therapy and patients with sterile urine should receive prophylactic antibiotics immediately prior to, and after, stent insertion.

Results

In a review of published data[14–24] on over 900 patients treated, approximately 70% of temporary prostatic stents achieve their objective, i.e. they remain in situ until the patient dies with a functioning stent or undergoes planned surgery. In addition there are now a significant number of patients, treated with a so-called temporary stent, who have had no complications from the stent for periods up to four years, or have had a new stent inserted at intervals rather than undergoing prostatic surgery. Significant complications associated with temporary stents, spiral coils or catheters are shown in Table 6.5. Proximal or distal migration may occur in up to 40% of patients but only requires stent removal in 7%. Similarly, short-term irritative symptoms will occur in up to 70% of men but are only severe and persistent in 5%.

Temporary stents are becoming less temporary and though considerably more expensive than a urethral catheter, they do appear to have significant advantages for the majority of men so treated.

Patients with long-term indwelling catheters are often physically disabled as a result of underlying chronic disease and place heavy demands on

Significant complications	Frequency (%)
Migration	7 ($\sim$ 40)*
Incontinence	6
Bacteriuria	4
Irritation	5 ($\sim$70)*
Pain	3
Bleeding	2
Obstruction	14
Infection	10
Encrustation	5

Table 6.5. Temporary prostatic stents/catheters
*See Results.

community and hospital resources because of the high incidence of catheter blockage, leakage, infection and haematuria. It is estimated that more than 50% of patients may suffer such problems[25] and over 90% will develop bacteriuria within four weeks.[26] In addition, little has been published on the psychological and sexual aspects of a permanent indwelling catheter.

More expensive metallic temporary stents do not appear to offer any significant advantages over the cheaper intraurethral catheters. Studies on the cost-effectiveness of such catheters in the treatment of bladder outflow obstruction, both in men who are fit and those considered unfit, are urgently required.

Stents in neurological voiding dysfunction

A combination of hyperreflexic detrusor function and external sphincter dyssynergia occurs in the majority of patients with suprasacral spinal cord injuries. Endoscopic sphincterotomy has been the treatment of choice but often has to be repeated and does not always ensure complete bladder emptying.

Indications for a stent

Patients with detrusor sphincter dyssynergia secondary to spinal cord injury who have failed previous endoscopic sphincterotomy.

Relative contraindications

There is little data on stent placement in these spinal injury patients and subsequent antegrade or retrograde ejaculation and future fertility. The presence of an artificial sphincter appears to be a contraindication if continence is a priority.

Results

The method of insertion is the same as for urethral strictures, except that a preliminary dilatation is not required. The results of 56 patients who have been treated with the first generation Urolume[TM] stent with a follow-up of 1–5 years have been published.[4,27,28] Complete voiding occurred in 47 patients. Seven stents were removed, 12 patients required additional stents and four a bladder-neck resection. The first publication on the use of a stent in patients with detrusor sphincter dyssynergia was by Shaw et al. in 1990.[4] It is surprising that, despite their initial success, there have been few additional reports as to the long-term value of this technique.[29]

Urethral strictures

Urethral strictures represent a common clinical urological problem and while urethral dilatation was once the mainstay of treatment, it has been largely superseded by endoscopic urethrotomy.

Cure rates attributed to visual urethrotomy in a meta-analysis of a number of series vary between 25 and 90% (mean 64%).[30] It is well recognized that there is a reduced chance of success following repeated urethrotomy. Reconstructive surgery is often complex and though producing excellent results for traumatic strictures, it is less successful for iatrogenic or infective strictures and there is a long-term recurrent stricture rate. Following urethrotomy the fibrotic area is disrupted and may be held open by long-term or intermittent catheterization. In 1987, following urethral dilatation, permanently implanted metal stents (Urolume[TM]) were inserted into the strictured area of patients with recurrent strictures irrespective of the aetiology to act as a scaffold during subsequent healing and thereby hopefully preventing restenosis of the urethra.[2] Both the titanium and the Memotherm[TM] stents have been used for the treatment of urethral strictures. However, the number of patients studied is small and there is no long-term follow-up.

More recently, a temporary implanted spiral of stainless steel, the Urocil (Instent USA), has been used.[31] In addition, Nissenkorn has recently described the use of a modified intraurethral catheter.[32]

Indications

Recurrent bulbar urethral strictures secondary to catheters or endoscopy.

Contraindications

Strictures in the penile shaft, transsphincteric strictures, traumatic strictures and strictures posturethroplasty.

Surgical technique

Urolume[TM] stent insertion

The majority of patients are treated under general anaesthesia in the lithotomy position. The stricture is dilated to at least 26 Fr and preferably

30 Fr. Alternatively, a triradiate optical urethrotomy is performed followed by the dilation. Urethrotomy should only be used in strictures which do not dilate easily as it may result in bleeding with difficulties in visualization at the time of stent insertion. A stent of appropriate length is chosen to cover the entire length of the stricture with a margin of normal urethra at either end. When implanted into the urethra the stent does not expand to its full extent. The stent is therefore correspondingly longer than in its unconstrained form. In the event of postoperative retention, a suprapubic catheter is inserted. Prophylactic antibiotic therapy is given prior to, and immediately following, stent insertion.

Urocoil insertion

The Urocoil (Instent USA) is inserted under fluoroscopic control. The proximal and distal ends of the stricture and the position of the external sphincter are marked by performing a urethrogram. The coil is inserted using either topical or regional anaesthesia. The stricture is either dilated or an internal urethrotomy performed and a coil, wound onto its delivery device, is passed 15–20 mm beyond the proximal end of the stricture. The stent is released from its introducing catheter and, as it does so, it expands and shortens approximately 25% of its length. The position of the stent can be checked using a small-calibre endoscope. Antibiotics are given for at least 5 days.

Insertion of the polyurethane urethral stent

This stent is a modification of the intraurethral catheter used for prostatic obstruction. It is 16 Fr in diameter and 30- or 40-mm long and is inserted through a 21 Fr urethrotome and positioned by pulling the 4.0 nylon thread connected to its distal end. A preliminary urethrotomy is performed and in the majority of patients this has been carried out under local anaesthesia.

Results

Urocoil[31]

Only short-term data are available on 18 patients. Four had mild dysuria and four stress incontinence corrected by readjusting the position of the coil. The mean follow-up was eight months. No encrustations were observed and pain was not a feature during an erection in those patients where the coil had been inserted into the penile urethra. The mean follow-up after removal of the stent in six patients is only five months. A recurrence of the stricture occurred in one.

Polyurethane urethral stent

Stents have been inserted into 22 patients using local anaesthetic. In 10, the stent was removed between three and five months and the strictures recurred in seven. It is now recommended that the stent is left in situ for at least 24 months. With the stent in situ all patients voided satisfactorily with a maximum flow varying between 17 and 23 ml/s. There were no reports of encrustation or obstruction of the stent.[32]

Urolume[TM] stent

There are two large multicentre studies, one from Europe and the other from the United States.[33,34] In the North American studies of stricture treatment[35] 175 patients with recurrent bulbar urethral strictures were studied. The mean peak flow had improved from 9.8 ± 6 ml/s to 22.4 ± 10 ml/s in the 95 patients available for study. Total symptom score had fallen from a mean of 12.7 pre-insertion to 2.3 at one year (range not given). The number of patients who underwent endoscopy at one year to assess epithelialization is also not stated but 88% of those that did had between 90 and 100% coverage. Untoward effects were mainly perineal discomfort, haematuria and postvoid dribbling (Table 6.6). Endourethral resection of hyperplastic urothelium was required in nine patients and 16 required the insertion of an additional stent. Five stents were removed. Postvoid dribbling appeared to be the only long-term untoward effect. In the European study,[33] 71 patients were treated with a follow-up of six months to two years. The complications seen were similar to that in the North American study. Endoscopy was performed in 31 cases. Epithelialization of the stent varied from 6 to 12 months and was slower in posturethroplasty strictures. The degree of hyperplasia within the stent also varied – in two cases the hyperplastic tissue had to be resected. With longer-term follow-up, hyperplasia and fibrous ingrowth have been reported. However, by limiting the use of the stent to recurrent strictures occurring as a result of endoscopy or catheterization, these stents should prove to be an acceptable method of treatment.

Conclusions

A role for permanently implanted stents in urethral strictures has now been defined. This is not the case, however, for the treament of bladder

Parameter	Mild	Moderate	Marked
Perineal discomfort (%)	13	3	1
Haematuria (%)	8	2	0
Postvoid dribble (%)	36	10	4
Discomfort with erection (%)	5	10	0

Table 6.6. Urethral stents (Urolume). North American experience (n = 95). Complications at 1 year (adapted from AMS Clinical Update, 1994)

Retreatment, n = 26. Removal, n = 5.

outflow obstruction. Permanently implanted stents are expensive and have not met with universal success. Both the Urolume^{TM}, Titan^{TM} and Memotherm^{TM} stents have had to undergo modifications from their original design. As a result the number of patients studied and the length of follow-up is short. There are no studies on the cost-effectiveness of these stents as an alternative to a prostatectomy.

Temporary stents for the treatment of bladder outflow obstruction have an overall success of around 70%. They are considerably cheaper than a permanent stent but more expensive than a urethral catheter. Studies on the cost-effectiveness of these stents as an alternative to prostatectomy or a long-term urethral catheter are urgently required. It is too early to draw any conclusions as to the role of a temporary stent in the management of urethral strictures.

References

1. Fabian KM. Der interprostatische 'partielle Katheter' (Urologische Spirale). Urologe 1980(A); 19: 236–8
2. Milroy EJG, Cooper JE, Wallsten H et al. A new treatment for urethral strictures. Lancet 1988; 1: 1424–7
3. Williams G, Jager R, McLoughlin J et al. Prostatic stents: a new treatment for prostatic outflow obstruction in patients unfit for surgery. BMJ 1989; 298: 1429
4. Shaw JPR, Milroy EJG, Timoney AG, Mitchel N. Permanent external sphincter stents in spinal injured patients. Br J Urol 1990; 66: 297–302
5. Williams G, Coulange C, Milroy EJ et al. The Urolume, a permanently implanted prostatic stent for patients at high risk for prostatic surgery. Br J Urol 1993; 72: 335–40
6. Guazzoni G, Montorsi F, Coulange C et al. A modified prostatic Urolume wallstent for healthy patients with symptomatic benign prostatic hyperplasia: A European Multicentre Study. Urology 1994; 44: 364–70
7. Bajoria S, Agarwal S, White R et al. Experience with the second generation Urolume prostatic stent. Br J Urol 1994; 75: 325–7
8. Kaplan SA, Merrill DC, Mosley WG et al. The titanium intraprostatic stent: the United States experience. J Urol 1993; 150: 1624–9
9. Miller PD, Gillet D, Kirby RS et al. The ASI titanium stent – 3 years experience. Paper presented at the 1992 Annual Meeting of BAUS, Bournemouth, UK
10. Holmes SAV, Miller PD, Crocker PR et al. Encrustation of intraoperative stents – a comparative study. Br J Urol 1992; 69: 383–7
11. ASI Clinical Update, May 1992
12. Abrams P, Gillat D, Chadwick D. Intraprostatic stent: experience with the ASI stent to treat bladder outflow obstruction (Abstract). J Urol 1991; 145: 293A
13. Parra RO. Titanium urethral stent an alternative to prostatectomy in the high risk surgical patients. J Urol 1991; 145: 293A
14. Nordling J, Poulsen AL. Prostatic stents: indications techniques and clinical results of the prostatic coil. In Fitzpatric JM (ed) Nonsurgical treatment of BPH. Edinburgh: Churchill Livingstone, 1992; 145–53
15. Harrison NW, deSouza JV. Prostatic stenting for outflow obstruction. Br J Urol 1990; 65: 192–6
16. Yachia D, Lask D, Rabinson S. Self retaining intraurethral stent an alternative to long term indwelling catheter or surgery in the treatment of prostatism. Am J Radiol 1990; 154: 111–13
17. Nielsen KK, Klarskov P, Nordling J et al. The intraprostatic spiral. New treatment for urinary retention. Br J Urol 1990; 65: 500–3
18. Billiet I, Mattelaer J, VanBrien P. Use of transrectal longitudinal sonography in the placement of a prostatic coil. Eur Urol 1990; 17: 76–8

19. Chevakier D, Quintens H, Amiel J et al. La spirale intra-prostatique dans le traitement de l'hypertrophie de la prostate. J d'Urologie 1990; 96: 203–6

20. Guazzoni G, Montorsi F, Columbo R et al. Long term experience with the prostatic spiral for urinary retention due to benign prostatic hyperplasia. Scand J Urol Nephrol 1991; 25: 21–4

21. Parker CJ, Birch BRP, Connelly A et al. The Porges urospiral: a reversible endoprostatic prosthetic stent. World J Urol 1991; 9: 22–5

22. Lewi H. The role of the intraprostatic spiral in 184 patients. Fifteen months follow up. Paper presented at the 1992 Annual Meeting of BAUS, Bournemouth, UK

23. Sassine AM, Schulman CC. Intraurethral catheter in high-risk patients with urinary retention: 3 years of experience. Eur Urol 1994; 25: 131–4

24. Yachia D, Beyar M, Aridogan IA. A new large calibre, self-expanding and self retaining temporary intraprostatic stent (Prostacoil) in the treatment of prostatic obstruction. Br J Urol 1994; 74: 47–9

25. Cools HJM, Van der Meer JWM. Restriction of long term urethral catheterization in the elderly. Br J Urol 1986; 58: 683–8

26. Slade N, Gillespie WA. The urinary tract and the catheter: infection and other problems. Chichester, Wiley, 1985; 11, 21, 35

27. McInerney PD, Vanner TF, Harris SAB, Stephenson TP. Permanent urethral stents for detrusor sphincter dyssynergia. Br J Urol 1991; 67: 291–4

28. Chancellor MB, Karusick S, Erhard MJ. Placement of a wire mesh prosthesis in the external urinary sphincter of men with spinal cord injuries. Radiology 1993; 187: 551–5

29. Chancellor MB, Ackman D, Aspell RA et al. Multicentre trials in N. America of Urolume urinary sphincter prosthesis. J Urol 1993; part 2 149, 358A. Abstract 580

30. Petersen NE. Traumatic posterior urethral avulsion. Monogr Urol 1986; 61–82

31. Yachia D, Beyar M. Temporarily implanted urethral coil stent for the treatment of recurrent urethral strictures: a preliminary report. J Urol 1991; 146: 1001–4

32. Nissenkorn I. A polyurethane urethral stent for the treatment of urethral strictures. Presented at the SIU Congress, Sydney, Australia, September 1994

33. Ashken MH, Coulange C, Milroy EJG, Sarramon JP. European experience with the urethral wallstent for urethral strictures. Eur Urol 1991; 19: 181–5

34. Oesterling JE, Defalco A and the North American Urolume Study Group: The Urolume endoprosthesis as a treatment for recurrent bulbar urethral strictures: long term results from the N. American Clinical Trial. J Urol 1993; part 2, 149, 505A. Abstract 1171

35. AMS Clinical Update – North American studies of stricture treatment, 1994

The artificial sphincter for treating male incontinence

7

D. M. Barrett E. Kleer

Introduction

The artificial urinary sphincter was introduced in 1973 as the AS721.[1] Since then the device has undergone a number of design modifications to improve its versatility and the overall degree of achieved continence. Equally important was the attempt to limit the incidence of device failure and postoperative complications. Two of the most clinically significant complications are recurrent incontinence caused by underlying urethral tissue atrophy and erosion of the cuff through the smooth muscle of the urethra.

The latest change in the AMS 800 was the introduction of the narrow-backed cuff design in June 1987 (Fig. 7.1(a) and (b)). The purpose of the design change was to improve the transmission of cuff pressure to the underlying tissue and to decrease the incidence of tissue pressure atrophy and cuff erosion. Also, it should be noted that since 1983 all cuffs have been incorporated with surface treatment, which theoretically should decrease the incidence of cuff erosion. The AMS 800 has become a valuable tool for the management of urinary incontinence in properly selected patients.

Preoperative evaluation

The incontinent patient most likely to benefit fom the implantation of an American Medical Systems 800 artificial genitourinary sphincter (AGUS) is the one with normal detrusor contractility and compliance associated with sphincteric incompetence. Typically this occurs with post prostatectomy incontinence. Patients with incontinence following trauma, radiation, or neurological disease are also likely to benefit from the implantation of an AGUS. Post prostatectomy incontinent patients obtain a 90–96% improved continence rate and a 90% satisfaction rate following implantation.[2,3] The preoperative evaluation prior to sphincter implantation should consist of a history, physical examination, urinalysis, urine Gram stain culture and sensitivity, urodynamics, radiologic imaging of the urinary tract, and urethrocystoscopy.

In patients with a history of post prostatectomy incontinence it is important to determine the length of time since the surgery, the severity of the incontinence in terms of pads worn per day (if it is improving, worsening, or stabilized) and the quality of the urinary stream. A minimum

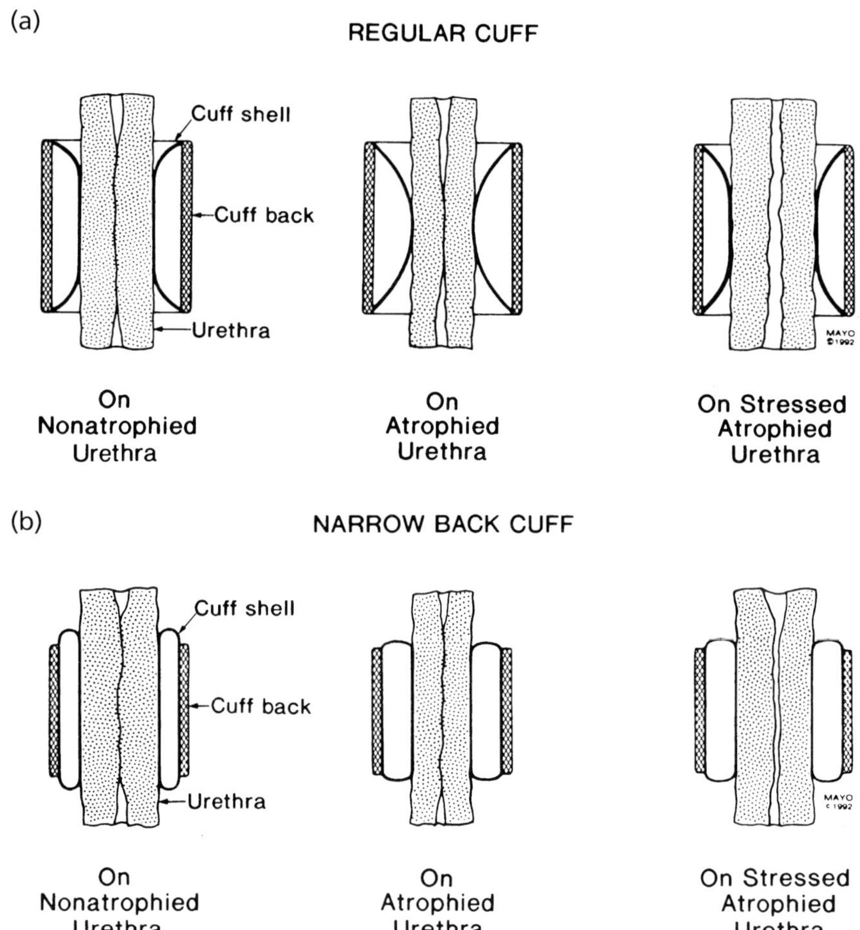

Fig. 7.1. (a) Dynamics of regular cuff of artificial urinary sphincter on nonatrophied, atrophied, and stress atrophied urethra showing non-uniform compression of urethral tissue. (b) Dynamics of recently designed narrow-backed cuff on nonatrophied, atrophied, and stressed atrophied urethra showing expansion of inner cuff along greater urethral length, allowing for more uniform compression of urethral tissue.

period of six months should be allowed between the time of prostatectomy and consideration of AGUS implantation as post prostatectomy incontinence can improve dramatically during this period of time. In addition it is important to ask if the patient has been on a regular program of pelvic strengthening exercises and if he has undergone a trial of pharmacologic therapy. Pelvic strengthening exercises and the use of anticholinergics and/or alphasympathomimetics may sometimes allow patients with minimal to mild incontinence to achieve a level of socially acceptable incontinence without resorting to surgery. A history of a dribbling flow of stream may give an indication as to the presence of a bladder neck contracture, urethral stricture, or meatal stenosis resulting in overflow incontinence. Patients with post prostatectomy strictures should be questioned regarding the number, frequency, and time of the last dilation. A history of strictures is not a contraindication to sphincter implantation unless they are located at the site where the cuff needs to be implanted. However, repeated urethral instrumentation in the presence of a sphincter may predispose the patient to cuff erosion.

It is also important to obtain a thorough history regarding strictures and their treatment in patients with a history of incontinence following radiation or trauma. Patients with a history of post traumatic urethral reconstruction are better served with placement of the cuff around the bladder neck whereas patients with a history of bladder neck reconstruction are better served with placement of the cuff around the bulbous urethra.

In patients with incontinence secondary to neurologic disease such as myelodysplasia, it is important to verify that a trial of pharmacologic treatment and intermittent catheterization have failed to enhance outlet resistance and/or increase bladder capacity to a point that results in socially acceptable incontinence. In patients with neurological disease it is recommended that the sphincter cuff is implanted around the bladder neck rather than the urethra as the result seems to be more physiologic.[4] Many of these patients require intermittent catheterization to completely empty their bladders. Catheter induced trauma is less likely to occur if the sphincter cuff is around the bladder neck rather than the bulbous urethra where the tissue is thinner and less well vascularized.

On physical examination many patients with chronic urinary incontinence have various degrees of dermatitis on the lower abdomen and pelvis. In these patients it is best to insert a Foley catheter several days prior to implantation to promote healing and reduce the possibility of infection. It is also important to look at the location of previous abdominal scars. It is preferable to implant the reservoir away from these scarred areas. Rectal examination should be performed to rule out recurrent cancer in post prostatectomy patients and for assessment of anal sphincter tone. Urinalysis, culture, and sensitivities are performed to assure urine sterility prior to AGUS implantation to minimize the likelihood of infection.

All patients with a history of neurologic disease should undergo intravenous pyelogram and voiding cystourethrogram to exclude upper tract or bladder structural abnormalities that would require repair prior to or during sphincter implantation.[4] Grade 2 reflux or greater should be corrected before or during sphincter implantation. Retrograde urethrograms are indicated in patients with a history of recurrent stricture, pelvic trauma, and/or urethral reconstruction.

Urodynamics is the next stage in evaluating whether the patient may be a candidate for sphincter implantation. Patients with detrusor instability and/or small capacity, poor complaint bladders are poor candidates for sphincter implantation. Pharmacologic agents or bladder augmentation may make such patients suitable candidates. The bladder must be able to hold volumes greater than 400 ml and maintain an intravesical pressure of less than 40 cmH$_2$O.[5]

Urethrocystoscopy is also necessary prior to implantation of an artificial sphincter to evaluate for false passages, strictures, contractures, diverticulae and foreign bodies. It is important to note the location of the urethral defect. For example, a stricture in the distal or midbulbous urethra may prevent implantation of the occlusive cuff at this level and an alternative site should be chosen. In post radiation patients cystoscopy is important to determine tissue viability prior to sphincter implantation to decrease the possibility of subsequent urethral erosion.[6]

Operative technique

Patients are admitted to the hospital on the morning of the surgical procedure. Those patients having bladder neck cuff placement should be instructed to have a limited lower bowel preparation the night prior to surgery. Parenteral broad spectrum antibiotics should be administered on-call to the operating room. Hair removal is done just prior to surgery. Patients undergoing the bladder neck cuff operation are positioned supine with their legs slightly abducted while those receiving the bulbous urethral cuff are positioned in the lithotomy position. A rectal tube is placed in patients who will have bladder neck cuff placement. A full ten-minute iodophor skin scrub should be performed. Draping should allow access to the lower anterior abdominal wall and perineum. A 12 French Foley catheter is subsequently inserted. An antibiotic solution should be available and used frequently for irrigation during the procedure.

Bladder neck cuff placement

A lower abdominal midline incision is made and carried down into the retropubic space. The dissection should be extraperitoneal as the peritoneal cavity does not need to be opened. Blunt dissection around the bladder neck is begun superior to the endopelvic fascia and inferior to a point where the ureters empty into the posterior aspect of the bladder. With the Foley catheter in place, the demarcation of the bladder neck and proximal portion of the urethra can be palpated. The plane is established between the posterior aspect of the bladder neck and the anterior surface of the rectum (Fig. 7.2). Palpation of the rectal tube may help in identifying the anterior surface of the rectum. Usually a combination of blunt and sharp dissection allows complete circumferential dissection. The width of this plane should be approximately 2 cm to allow unrestricted placement of the cuff. A tape is passed around the bladder neck, and the bladder is filled with antibiotic solution to reveal any small tears that may have been

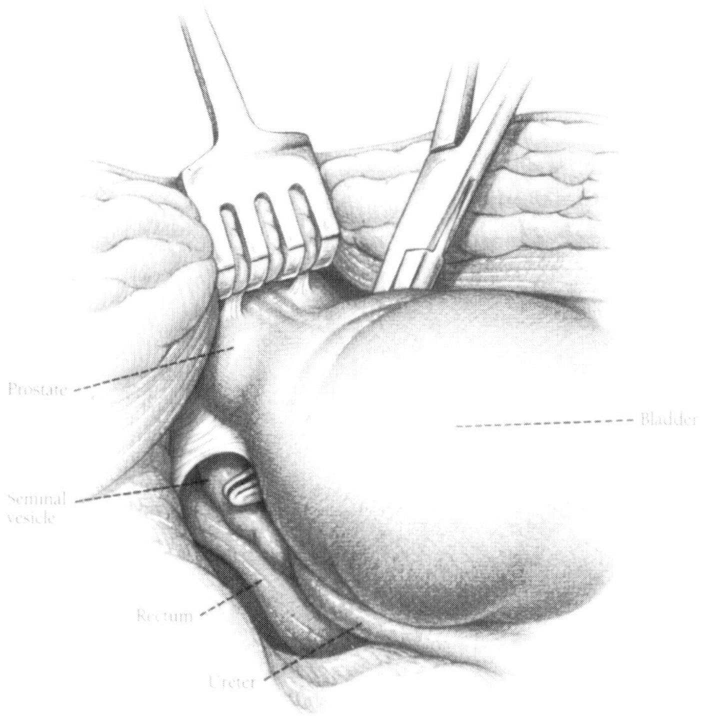

Fig. 7.2. Blunt dissection of the bladder neck. The plane is established between the posterior aspect of the bladder neck and the anterior surface of the rectum. Dissection is begun superior to the endopelvic fascia but inferior to a point where the ureters empty into the posterior aspect of the bladder. From Barrett DM. Implantation of an artificial sphincter. In Barrett DM ed, Urologic Surgery. Learning Technology Inc., New Scotland, NY, 1988.

created during the dissection. If present, they may be closed with 3-0 or 4-0 absorbable sutures. However, if a rectal injury is identified it should be closed primarily and the procedure abandoned for a later date. The bladder neck is circumferentially measured with the calibrated measuring strap (Fig. 7.3). The indwelling Foley catheter need not be removed prior to this measurement unless it is greater than 12 French. In men, an 8 to 14 cm cuff may be necessary. The properly sized cuff is then passed underneath the bladder neck and snapped in place (Fig. 7.4). The tubing from the cuff is then passed through the belly of one rectus muscle and through the anterior abdominal wall fascia on the side of the patient where the pump will be placed. The tubing from the cuff should penetrate the rectus muscle and fascia and into the deep subcutaneous tissues from 7 to 10 cm above the pubic symphysis. A curved shod clamp is used on the end of the cuff tubing closed with only one click.

The pressure balloon reservoir is placed in the prevesical space. Its tubing penetrates the rectus muscle next to the tubing of the cuff. A straight shod clamp closed with only one click is left on the end of the

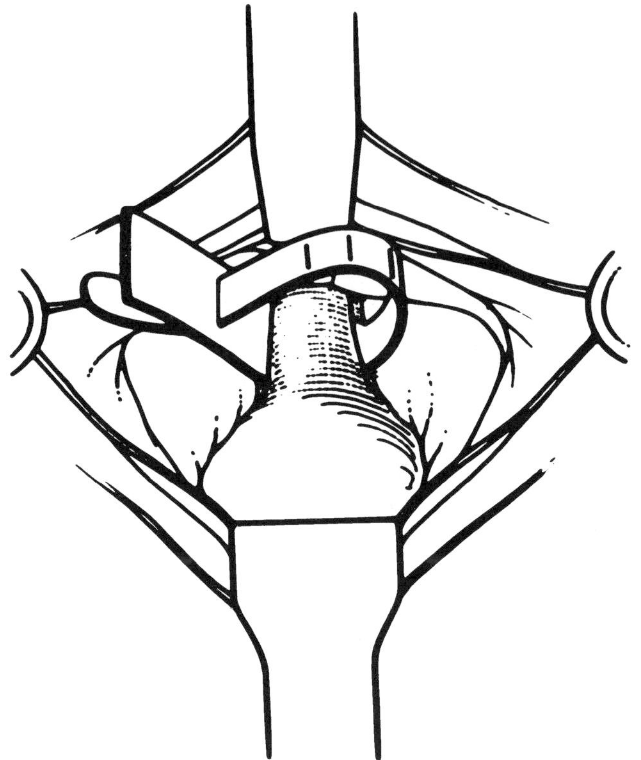

Fig. 7.3. The bladder neck is circumferentially measured with the calibrated measuring strap. The bladder neck must be circumferentially dissected. The width of the plane should be approximately 2 cm to allow unrestricted placement of the cuff. (Courtesy of American Medical Systems, Inc., Minnetonka, MN.)

reservoir tubing (Fig. 7.5). Before the balloon is filled the prevesical space is drained and the anterior abdominal wall fascia is closed with absorbable suture. After completion of the closure the balloon is filled with 22 ml of iso-osmotic contrast medium. A 61–70 cmH$_2$O pressure balloon reservoir is routinely used in most patients. Using a Hegar dilator a lateral hemiscrotal pocket is developed for the control assembly (Fig. 7.5). The pump is placed in an optimally dependent position with the activation/deactivation button laterally, easily palpable against the skin (Fig. 7.6(a)-(b)). A curved shod clamp should be on the control tubing to the cuff and a straight shod clamp on the control tubing to the reservoir, each closed with only one click. Appropriate connections are made between the sphincter components using straight connectors tied in place with 2-0 prolene suture (Fig. 7.7). Connections may also be made with the quick-connect connectors. The incision is closed in layers with absorbable suture. After the device has been tested and cycled the cuff is left in an open deactivated position.

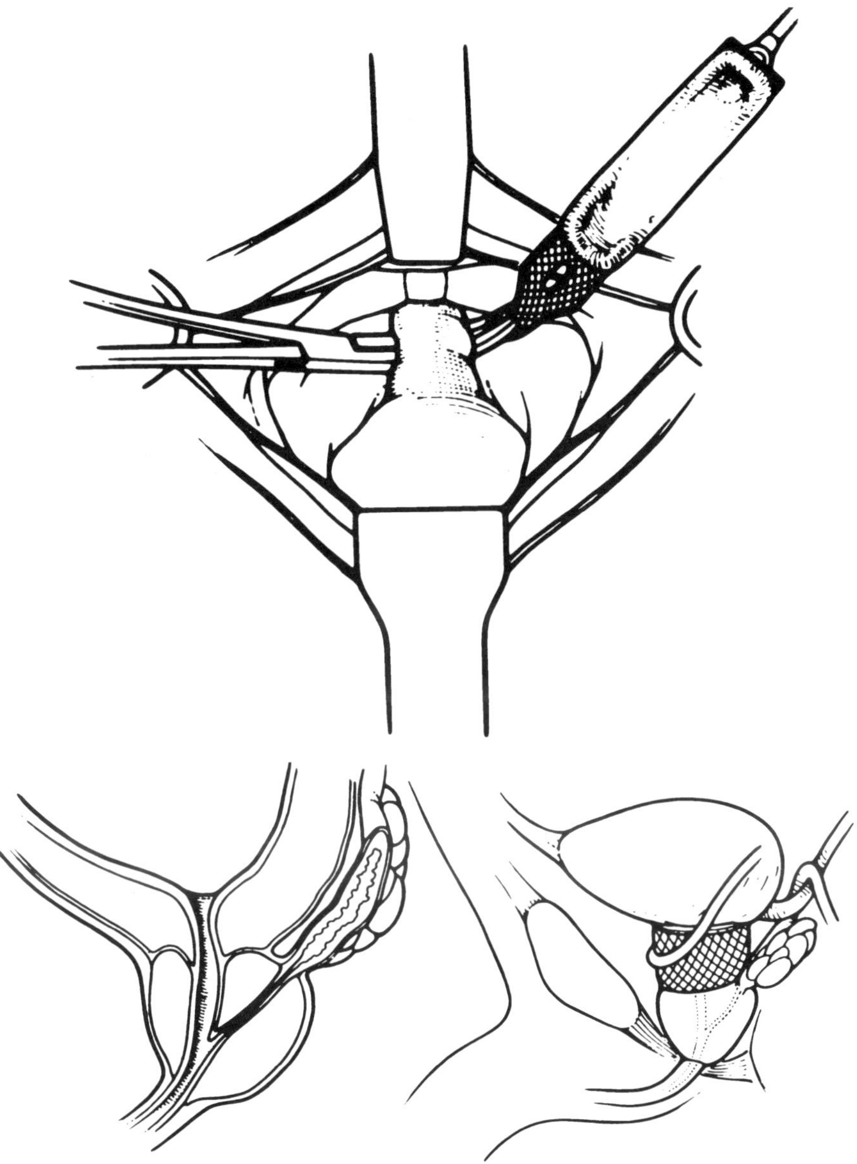

Fig. 7.4. The properly sized cuff is passed underneath the bladder neck and strapped in place while gentle opposing traction is applied to the tab and tubing. Care should be made that the tubing attached to the cuff is directed towards the side where the pump and reservoir will be inserted. (Courtesy of American Medical Systems, Inc., Minnetonka, MN.)

As discussed earlier, those patients with detrusor instability and/or small capacity, poor-compliant bladders may require concomitant bladder augmentation intestinocystoplasty at the time of sphincter implantation.

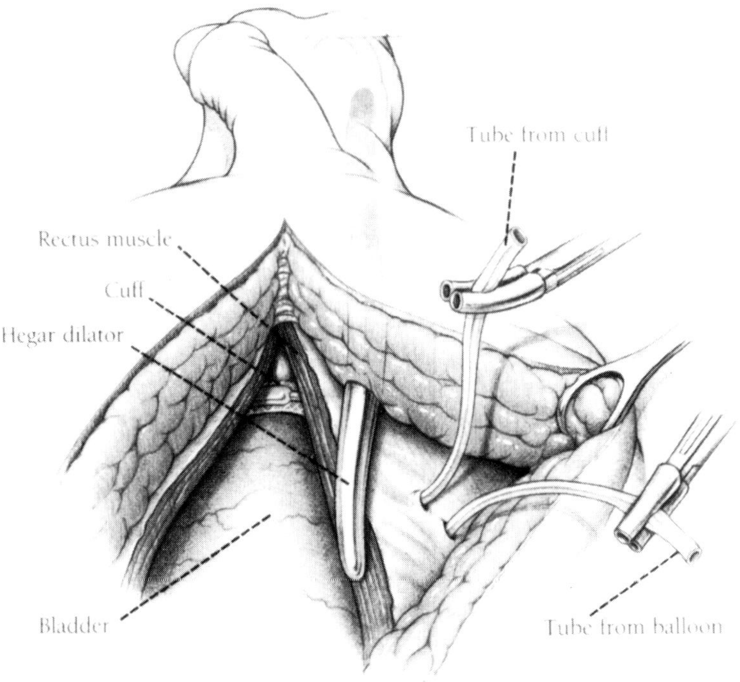

Fig. 7.5. After the cuff and reservoir tubes are brought through the rectus muscle, a Hegar dilator is used to create a deep pocket through the subcutaneous tissues, above Scarpa's fascia into the right hemiscrotum. The control assembly will be placed in this pocket. From Barrett DM. In Barrett DM Ed, Urologic Surgery. Learning Technology Inc., New Scotland, NY, 1988.

The cuff should be placed around the bladder neck when possible since many of these patients will require clean intermittent catheterization (Fig. 7.8).[7] The augmentation cystoplasty should be completed prior to insertion of the sphincter. Ample space should be allowed around the bladder neck area for the cuff to be placed without impinging on any of the suture lines.

Bulbous urethral cuff

A small perineal incision is made over the bulbous urethra (Fig. 7.9). With a Young retractor superiorly and a Gillespie retractor for lateral exposure, the bulbous urethra is dissected circumferentially (Fig. 7.10). If possible, dissection should be carried out around the bulbocavernosus muscle and a plane established between it and the tunica albuginea of the corporal bodies. This plane allows the cuff to be placed around the bulbocavernosus muscle and not directly on the bulb of the urethra to reduce the risk of erosion. The width of this dissection must be adequate to accommodate the 2 cm width of the cuff. Care is taken not to injure the urethra at the 12 o'clock position, the point at which dissection is most

(a)

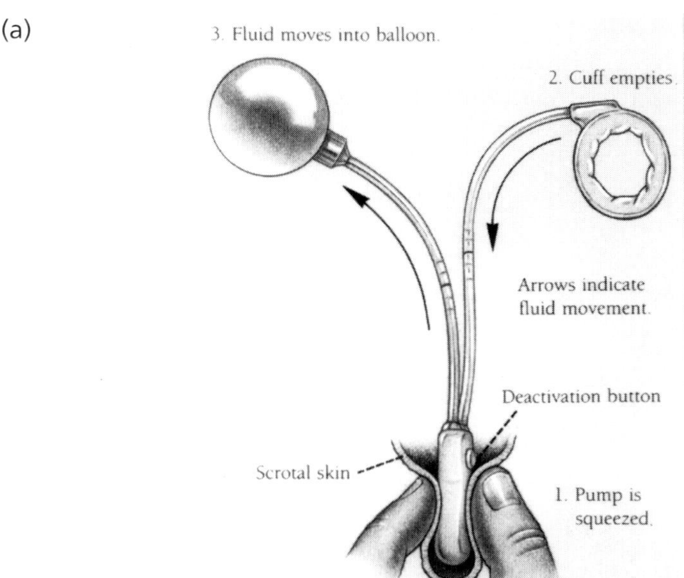

(b)

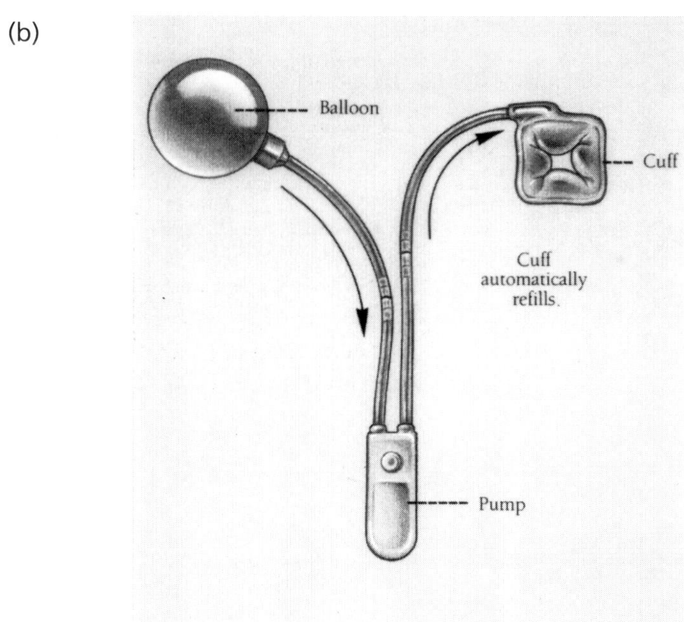

Fig. 7.6. (a) *The pump is placed in an optimally dependent position with the activation/deactivation button laterally. This button must be easily palpable against the scrotal skin. To void, the patient squeezes the pump through the scrotal skin. (b) When the patient stops squeezing the pump the cuff will begin to refill automatically. From Barrett DM. Implantation of an artificial sphincter. In Barrett DM ed, Urologic Surgery. Learning Technology Inc., New Scotland, NY, 1988.*

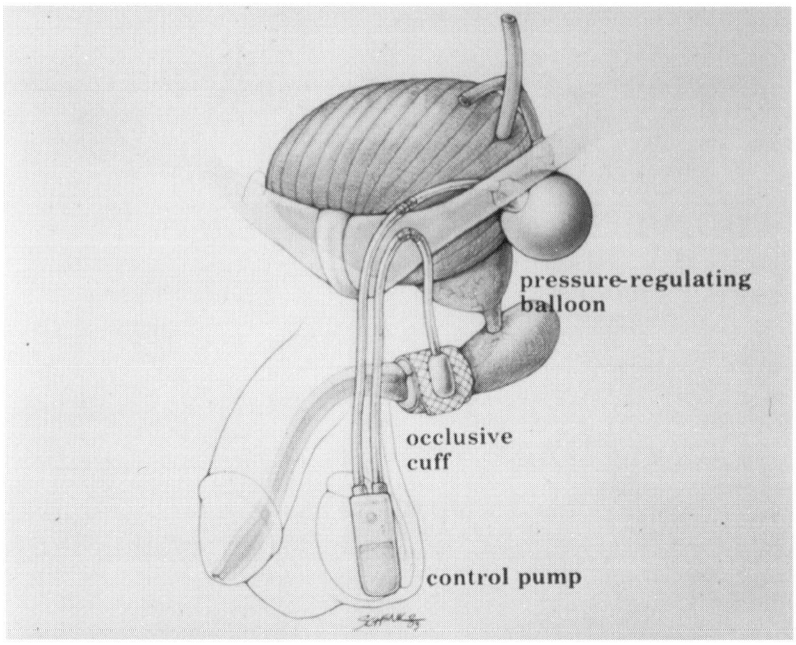

Fig. 7.7. The implantation of the artificial genitourinary sphincter with a bladder neck cuff has been completed.

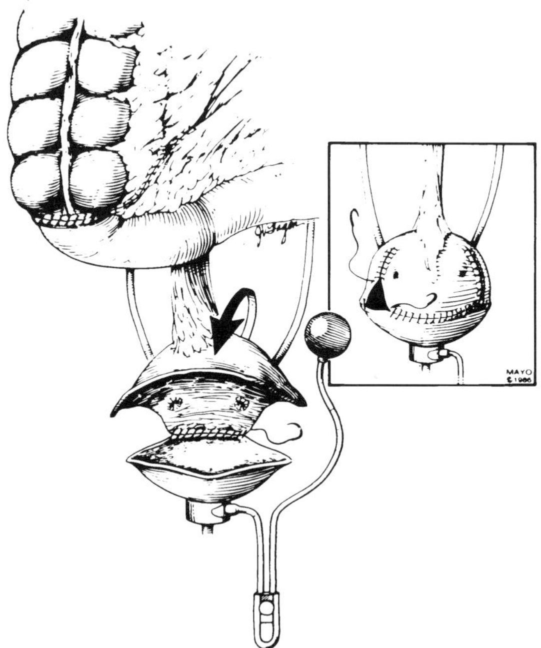

Fig. 7.8. When performing bladder augmentation intestinocystoplasty concommitantly with sphincter implantation the cuff should be placed around the bladder neck when possible. The cuff should not be impinging of any of the suture lines. (With permission of Mayo Foundation.)

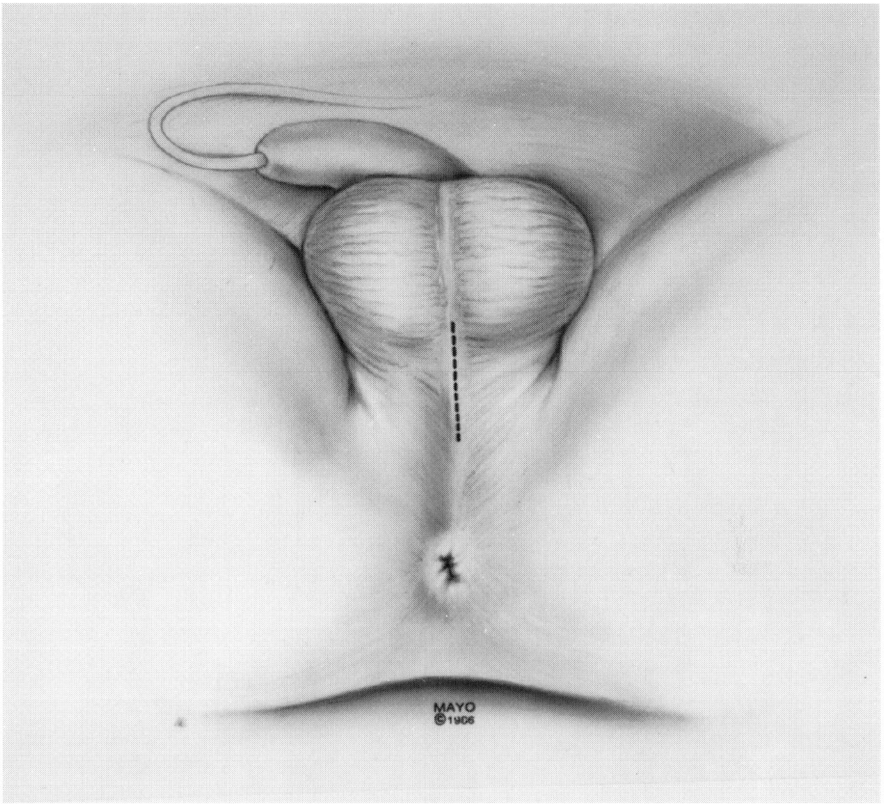

Fig. 7.9. With a Foley catheter in place a small perineal incision is made over the bulbous urethra. (Courtesy of Mayo Foundation.)

difficult and most urethral injuries occur. If the urethra is injured it may be possible to close the defect primarily with 4-0 or 5-0 absorbable suture. A different site on the urethra can then be selected for cuff placement. Routinely a 4.5 cm cuff is passed tab first beneath the urethra (Fig. 7.11) and the cuff is snapped into place while gentle opposing traction is applied to the tab and tubing. Care should be made that the tubing attached to the cuff is directed towards the side where the pump and reservoir will be inserted. A curved shod clamp closed with only one click is placed around the cuff tubing for later identification.

Subsequently a small transverse incision is made in the lower abdominal wall to the side where the pump and reservoir will be located. In general this should be the side of hand dominance. After the anterior fascia is exposed it is vertically incised for a short distance and a pocket is bluntly developed below the belly of the rectus muscle, extraperitoneally, to allow placement of the deflated balloon reservoir (Fig. 7.12). The reservoir tubing is brought through a separate stab incision in the anterior rectus fascia. The reservoir is subsequently filled with 22 ml of iso-osmotic

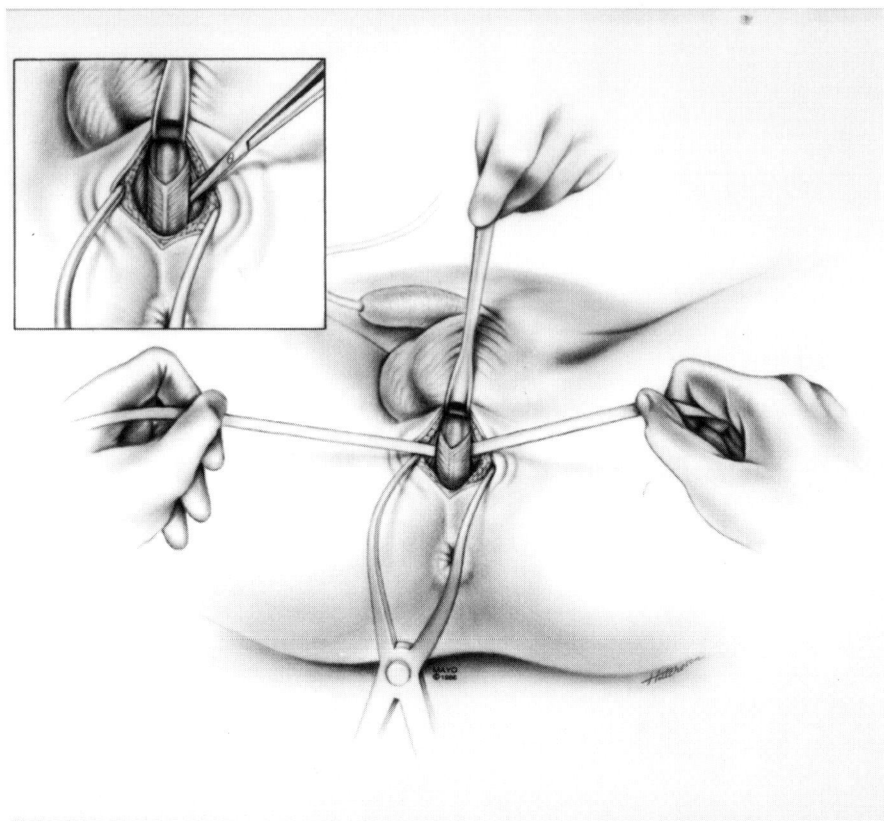

Fig. 7.10. With a Young retractor superiorly and a Gillespie retractor for lateral exposure the bulbous urethra has been circumferentially dissected. The width of this dissection must be able to accommodate the 2 cm width of the cuff. Inset. Sharp dissection is used to enter a plane between the bulbocavernosal muscle and the tunica albuginea of the corporal bodies to gain circumferential access. (With permission of Mayo Foundation.)

contrast medium and a straight shod clamp is placed around the tubing and closed with only one click to prevent fluid loss. A 61–70 cmH$_2$O pressure balloon reservoir is routinely used in most patients with uncomplicated bulbous urethral cuffs. In high risk patients the 51–60 cmH$_2$O pressure balloon reservoir is used to minimize tissue pressure ischemia. After assuring that the inflated balloon is well accommodated with the rectus pocket, the fascial defect is closed with a running absorbable suture.

A long clamp is then passed from the plane superior to the rectus fascia, above Scarpa's fascia, to the area of the perineal incision (Fig. 7.11). The cuff tubing is grasped and guided to the area of the lower quadrant incision. Next, a lateral subcutaneous hemiscrotal pouch is created with Hegar dilators where the pump is placed in an optimally dependent position with the activation/deactivation button laterally (Figs 7.5 and 7.6). The activation/deactivation button must be easily palpable against the skin.

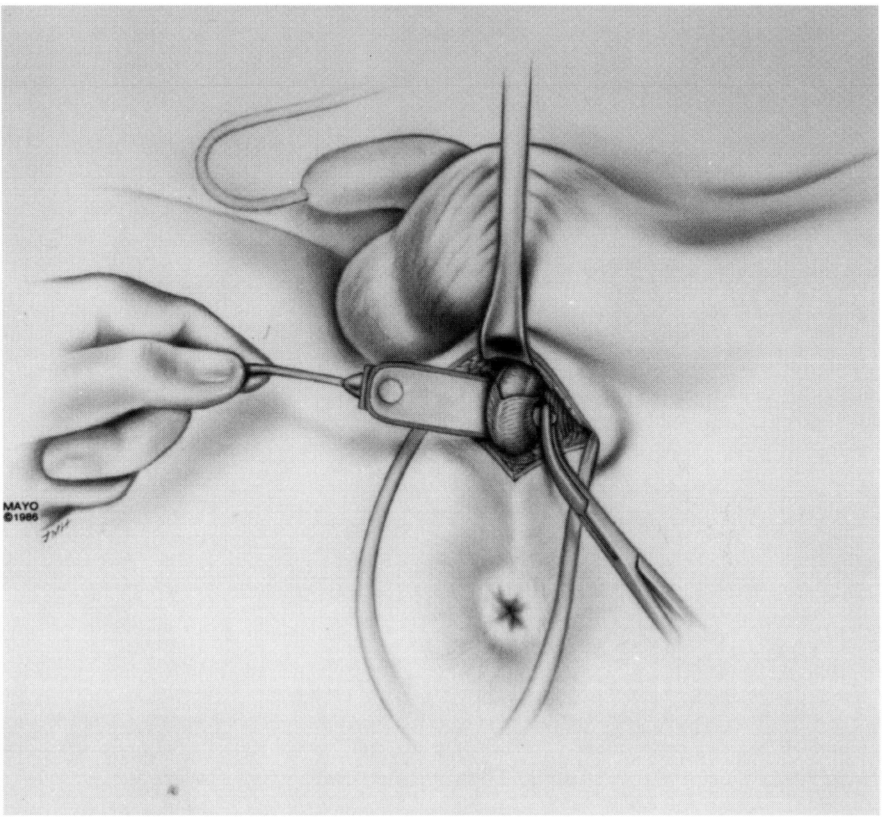

Fig. 7.11. Routinely a 4.5 cm cuff is passed tab-first beneath the urethra. It is snapped in place while gentle opposing traction is applied to tab and tubing. The tubing should be directed toward the side where the pump and reservoir will be inserted. (With permission of Mayo Foundation.)

Once a satifactory position for the pump has been assured a Babcock clamp is placed around it and the scrotal skin to prevent its proximal migration when the tubing is connected. The pump tubing that will be connected to the cuff tubing should have a curved shod clamp around it while a straight shod clamp should be placed around the other tubing which will be connected to the reservoir tubing.

All of the appropriate tubing connections are then made (Fig. 7.13). The cuff tubing is attached to the control assembly tubing with a right-angle connector to prevent kinking. The balloon and the control assembly tubing are attached with a straight connector. These connectors can be tied in place with 2-0 prolene or they may be assembled with the quick-connect tubing connections.

The incisions are closed in layers with absorbable suture and the sphincter is left in a cuff-open deactivated position after the device has been tested and cycled. Pressure dressings are applied.

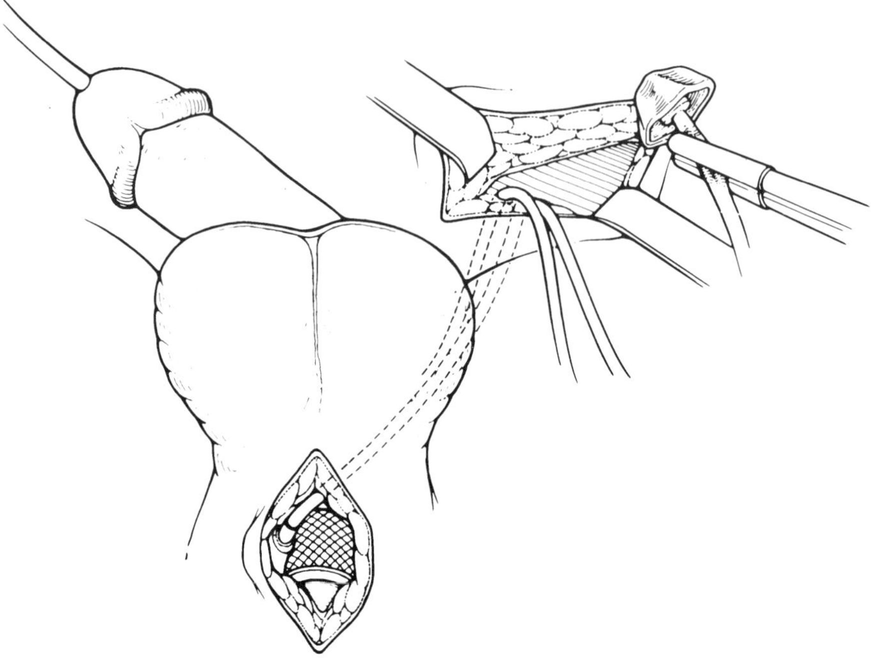

Fig. 7.12. The deflated balloon reservoir is placed in a pocket below the belly of the rectus muscle. The cuff tubing has been guided to this area through the subcutaneous tissues. (Courtesy of American Medical Systems, Inc., Minnetonka, MN.)

Postoperative management

The Foley catheter is removed the following day. The patient should have ice packs applied to the scrotum and/or perineum for the first 24 hours postoperatively to minimize edema and hematoma formation. Some patients experience a transient postoperative continence secondary to tissue edema around the cuff site. Once the incontinence reoccurs, the patient is advised to use pads or condom drainage devices. The use of penile clamps is discouraged. In the rare instances in which the patient is unable to urinate, self intermittent catheterization with a small caliber catheter should be instituted.

Activation of the sphincter is performed six to eight weeks postoperatively. Activation is performed by firm compression of the pump. The deactivation button will switch into the activated configuration, allowing fluid to circulate through the control assembly. Activation can be monitored by deflate and inflate radiographs which confirm filling of the cuff after activation. During this clinic visit patient reeducation regarding the sphincter operation is beneficial.

Patients who are dry at night in a recumbent position are instructed to deactivate their sphincter prior to falling asleep. This reduces the risk of

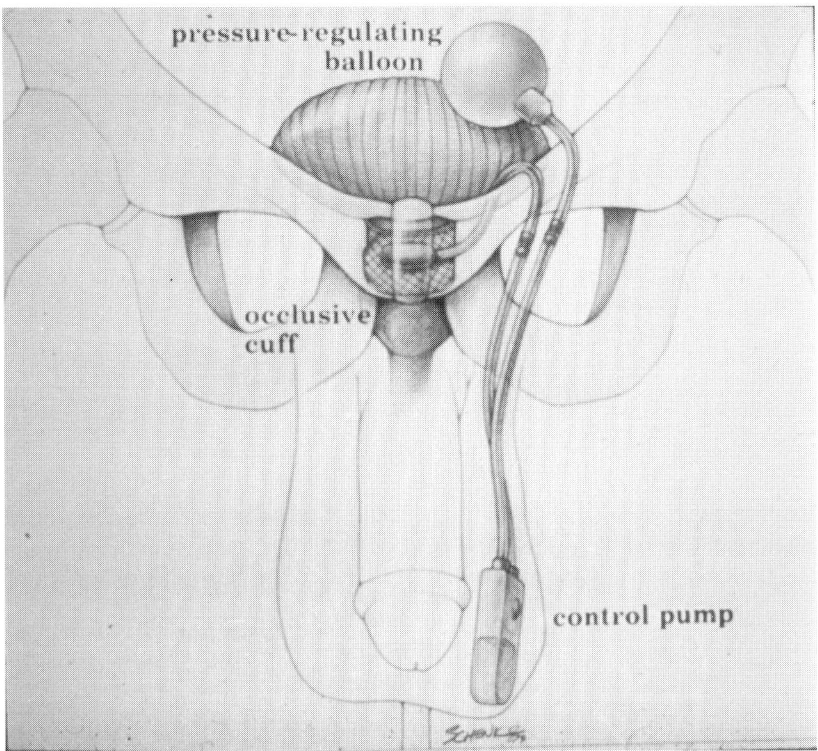

Fig. 7.13. The implantation of the artificial sphincter with a bulbar urethral cuff has been completed. From Barrett DM, Furlow WL, Goldwasser B. The artificial sphincter. In Yalla SV, McGuire EJ, Elbadawi A, Blaivas JG eds, Neurology and urodynamics: principles and practice. McGraw-Hill, Inc., New York, NY, 474–488, 1988.

ischemia to the underlying urethra or bladder neck. Patients who have diminished flow rates may require a second pumping to allow enough time to adequately empty their bladder before cuff recompression occurs. Patients unable to completely empty their bladders such as those with neurogenic bladders or bladder augmentations should use self intermittent catheterization. The sphincter cuff must be deflated prior to catheter insertion into the bladder.

Postoperative complications

Hematoma formation is the most common minor complication of sphincter implantation. It has the potential to displace the pump into an unfavorable location for external manipulation. A large hematoma may need to be drained to prevent discomfort and enhance healing.

Cuff erosion is most common in the first three to four months after implantation. Its incidence has decreased dramatically with 3 of 144 patients in a recent series since the introduction of the AMS 800 narrow-backed cuff design.[8] Cuff erosion prior to activation implies an unrecognized iatrogenic injury to the urethra or bladder neck. Cuff erosion may present as pain or swelling in the cuff or pump area, recurrent incontinence, urethral discharge, and/or urosepsis. Retrograde urethrography and urethroscopy confirm the diagnosis. Surgical removal of the cuff is mandatory. The remaining sphincter components should be removed if there is also purulent drainage. If the erosion is clean and uncomplicated only the cuff needs to be removed and a stainless steel plug is used to temporarily occlude the tube leading to the pump. Copious irrigation of the surrounding area with antibiotic solution and drainage may prevent subsequent infection around the device components. For bulbar urethral erosions a 12 or 14 French catheter is left indwelling. For bladder neck erosions an 18 French silicone catheter should be left indwelling for two to four weeks or until the retrograde urethrogram is normal.

Once complete healing occurs and if there is no evidence of infection a new cuff may be inserted. Bladder neck cuff replacement is facilitated if at the time of cuff removal the eroded opening is closed with absorbable sutured and a thin silicone strip is placed around the bladder neck. This facilitates reoperation and cuff replacement by the plane maintained by the silicone strip. On the other hand, if infection cannot be ruled out at the time of cuff removal then the peritoneum should be opened and an omental wrap should be positioned around the bladder neck to facilitate redissection. Despite these precautionary measures the patient should be forewarned that bladder neck cuff reimplantation may be impossible. In the case of a urethral cuff another location around the bulbar urethra should be selected for reimplantation.

In cases of infected sphincter components the entire device should be removed and the wound should be copiously irrigated and drained. Reimplantation may be considered at a later date.

Recurrent urinary incontinence following successful sphincter implantation requires a systematic approach to identify the problem.[9,10] The control assembly should be checked to be sure that it is in the activated state. If an inflate/deflate film is normal cystoscopy should be performed to rule out an erosion. Mechanical malfunction may result from fluid leakage, tube kinks and disconnections, and control pump malfunction. The most common site of fluid leakage is the cuff. Another potential site of mechanical failure is occlusion of the control assembly secondary to debris. Urodynamics should be performed to evaluate for detrusor hyperreflexia. Incontinence post artificial sphincter implantation may also result from suboptimal occlusive pressure secondary to urethral atrophy or suboptimal occlusive cuff pressure. Reduction in cuff size is an option for compensation of recurrent or persistent incontinence in a patient with an otherwise normally functioning sphincter. In patients with bladder neck cuffs the dissection of the implanted cuff is more difficult and thus it is recommended that an attempt be made to raise the balloon pressure initially. Sometimes results may also be improved with pharmacological agents which decrease detrusor contactility or enhance outlet resistance.

Patients with neurologic disorders such as myelomeningocele who have undergone sphincter implantation may be at risk for developing upper tract deterioration secondary to high voiding pressures and this require regular follow-up. This should consist of an excretory urogram or ultrasonographic assessment of the kidneys and urodynamic evaluation beginning within the first three to six months postoperatively. Should hydronephrosis develop the treatment is based on decreasing detrusor pressure and may be accomplished by increasing the frequency of intermittent catheterization, anticholinergics, and bladder augmentation if needed.

References

1. Scott FB, Bradley WE, Timm GW. Treatment of urinary incontinence by implantable prosthetic sphincter. Urology 1973; 1: 252
2. Gundian JC, Barrett DM, Parulkar BG. Mayo Clinic experience with use of the AMS 800 artificial urinary sphincter for urinary incontinence following radical prostatectomy. J Urol 1989; 142: 1459
3. Gundian JC, Barrett DM, Parulkar BG. Mayo Clinic experience with use of the AMS 800 artificial urinary sphincter for urinary incontinence after transurethral resection of prostate or open prostatectomy. Urology 1993; 41: 318
4. Barrett DM, Goldwasser B. The artificial urinary sphincter: current management philosophy. American Urological Association Updates 1986; Vol 5, Lesson 32
5. Petrou SP, Barrett DM. The expanded role for the artificial sphincter. American Urological Association Updates 1991; Vol 10, Lesson 16
6. Light JK. Implantation of the AS800 artificial urinary sphincter. Problems in Urology 1993; 7: 402
7. Strawbridge LR, Kramer SA, Castilla OA, *et al.* Augmentation cystoplasty and the artificial genitourinary sphincter. J Urol 1989; 142: 297
8. Leo ME, Barrett DM. Success of the narrow-backed cuff design of the AMS 800 artificial urinary sphincter: analysis of 144 patients. J Urol 1993; 150: 1412
9. Furlow WL, Barrett DM. Recurrent or persistent urinary incontinence in patients with the artificial urinary sphincter: diagnostic considerations and management. J Urol 1985; 133: 792
10. Marks JL, Light JK. Management of urinary incontinence after prostatectomy with the artificial urinary sphincter. J Urol 1989; 142: 302

Artificial urinary sphincters in the treatment of non-neurogenic female urinary incontinence

8

B. J. Norlén

Introduction

Female urinary incontinence is a common disorder and negatively affects the quality of life of many women. The condition has important consequences for health services and for health-care costs. In addition, severe urinary incontinence is a personal tragedy for many patients. In most cases, female urinary incontinence is 'simple stress incontinence', which can be treated successfully with different colposuspension or sling procedures. However, in true sphincteric incompetence, where traditional surgery has failed, and in congenital anomalies, placement of an artificial urinary sphincter might be the only solution to an extremely difficult problem. In such cases, placement of an artificial urinary sphincter is an alternative to urinary diversion. In the previous chapter, the history and development of artificial urinary sphincters is explained and their function described. The surgical procedure for placement of the device in males is covered in detail. In the female, the bladder neck must be widely exposed for cuff placement. An infected device is a major problem and all measures to minimize the risk of nosocomial infections must be taken.

Surgical procedure

Preparation of the patient

In order to avoid infection, at least one negative urine culture should be obtained prior to surgery. Urinary-tract infection should be treated for at least one week prior to surgery. Instrumentation of the urinary tract should be avoided within the 48 hours prior to surgery. The patient is encouraged to take a shower with chlorhexidine soap the night before surgery and on the morning of the day of surgery. Single infusions of prophylactic antibiotics (1.5 g cefpirom and 1 g vancomycin) are administered 1 hour before surgery so that a peak concentration is attained at the start of surgery. Hair shaving is delayed until the patient is on the operating table and thus done immediately prior to surgery. A thorough scrubbing of the skin for 10 min and a careful vaginal sterilization are undertaken before draping.

Positioning of the patient

A good exposure of the bladder neck with the possibility of manipulating the vagina and undertaking a cystoscopy are essential. These goals can be achieved by positioning the patient on low crutches with the thighs abduced but only slightly flexed.

Placement of artificial sphincter

A low transverse abdominal incision with a transsection of the rectus abdominis muscles provides an excellent exposure of the bladder neck area (Fig. 8.1A–C)[1]. The perivesical space is entered. In patients subjected to previous surgery, this retropubic dissection can be extremely difficult. Placement of a Foley catheter in the urethra with the balloon at the bladder neck area facilitates the identification of these structures. The endopelvic fascia is entered lateral to the bladder neck. A finger in the vagina is helpful in identifying the appropriate plane of dissection between

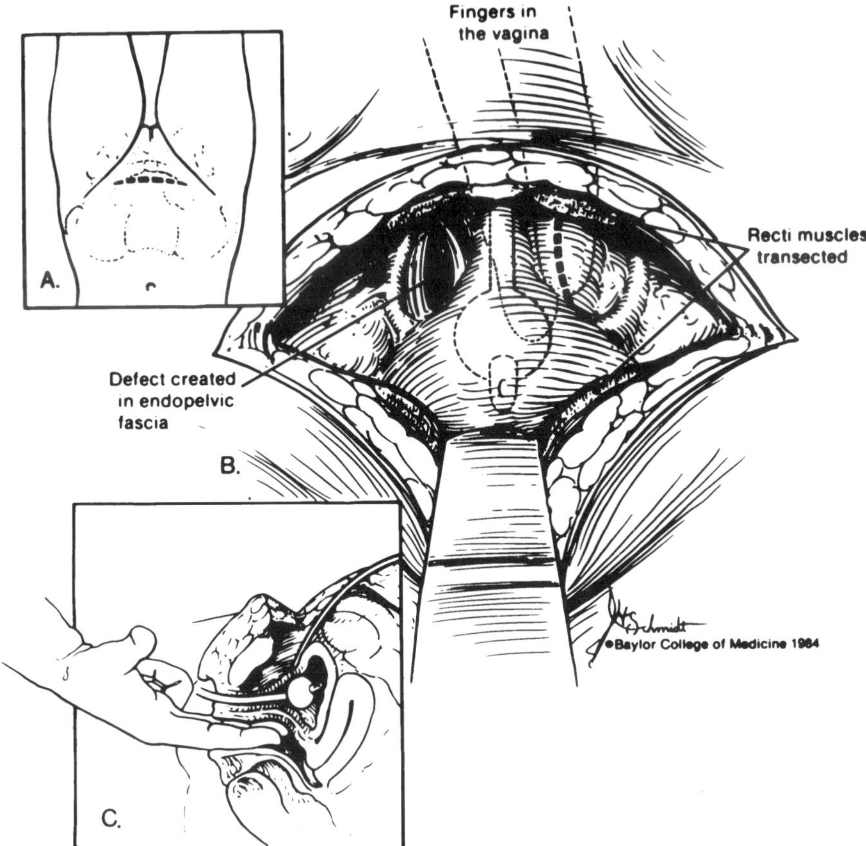

Fig. 8.1. Surgical technique for implantation of the artificial urinary sphincter in the female. From: Clin Obstet Gynecol 1985; 12:2, with permission from WB Saunders.

the bladder neck and the vaginal wall. With scissors, dissection is performed on each side of the bladder neck against the finger in the vagina and continued until the vaginal wall is reached. If uncertainty exists concerning the position of these structures, the bladder can be opened away from the area of planned cuff placement. The dissection behind the urethra and bladder neck through the urethorvaginal septum is crucial since perforation of the urethra or extensive dissection leaving a poorly vascularized tissue under the cuff will predispose for future cuff erosion. The passage must allow the placement of the cuff which is 2-cm wide. The length of the cuff is estimated with the help of a measuring tape. The tube of the cuff is then passed through the abdominal wall with a tubing needle. The balloon is placed in the perivesical space and the pump is placed in the greater labium. In the majority of cases, a balloon with a pressure range of 61–70 cmH$_2$O is chosen. For cuff lengths greater than 7–8 cm and in young, physically active women, a higher pressure range could be considered. A balloon with a lower pressure is chosen if the tissue underlying the cuff is of poor quality, i.e. after radiotherapy. The tubings are connected outside the abdominal wall after the different components have been fitted according to the instructions of the manufacturer. The device is inactivated until tenderness and swelling subside and allow a comfortable manipulation of the pump. The surgical incisions are closed with absorbable sutures. Drains can generally be avoided.

Indications (Table 8.1)

Patients falling into this category are those with a true sphincteric incompetence. The most common group is made up of patients with antistress incontinence surgery failures. Other important conditions are patients with congenital anomalies, such a congenitally short urethras and epispadias. Incontinence following pelvic trauma, i.e. pelvic fractures, and urethral surgery are also conditions suitable for treatment with an artificial sphincter.

- Failed antistress incontinence surgery
- Congenital anomalies
- Pelvic trauma
- Urethral surgery

Table 8.1. Indications for artificial urinary sphincter in non-neurogenic female incontinence.

Work-up of candidates for artificial urinary sphincter (Table 8.2)

An intravenous pyelography is mandatory in order to exclude upper-tract dilation, stones and anomalies. A micturition cystography will reveal reflux, a condition that can generally be corrected with re-implantation of the refluxing ureter at the time of sphincter placement. A urodynamic investigation will reveal any detrusor instability, a condition often associated with incontinence in women and one which might convert the placement of an artificial urinary sphincter into a failure. The urodynamic investigation will also evaluate the compliance of the bladder wall and the urethral closure pressure. In Barrett's experience, a decreased compliance expressed as an increase in pressure exceeding 15 cmH$_2$O per 100 cc volume infused indicates the need for an augmentation cystoplasty[2]. Sand and co-workers[3] found a urethral closure pressure of less than 20 cmH$_2$O to be a high risk of surgical failure with the Burch colposuspension procedure.

Urography
- Upper tract dilation

Urodynamic investigation
- Detrusor instability
- Bladder compliance
- Urethral closure pressure

Micturition cytography
- Reflux

Table 8.2. Work-up.

Patient selection (Table 8.3)

A careful evaluation of the patient and of the family situation for children is essential to avoid serious complications with the artificial urinary sphincter (AUS)[4]. The patient receiving an AUS must be highly motivated to manipulate the device and also aware of the possible need for clean intermittent catheterization. Besides motivation, the candidate for AUS needs to be of normal intelligence and also have a manual dexterity appropriate for handling the device and for undertaking clean intermittent catheterization.

Personal
- Motivation
- Intelligence
- Manual dexterity

High risk?
- Previous sling surgery
- Radiotherapy

Table 8.3. Patient selection.

Patients with a high risk of complications should be identified and, for patients with previous sling surgery and radiotherapy, the failure rate in most series is above 50%; for this reason, placement of an AUS should be avoided in these two categories[5].

Results

The main category of women who receive artificial sphincters for incontinence are those with a neurogenic bladder dysfunction. In the published literature, most series on non-neurogenic urinary incontinence treated with artificial sphincters are small or difficult to assess since they are combined with other aetiologies. Some results are summarized in Table 8.4. As can be seen, the results for patients with non-neurogenic incontinence are extremely good with a success rate of approximately 90%. It must be noted, however, that the revision rate, due to various reasons, in many materials is very high, viz. 20–50%. The most common causes for revision in Schreiter's large series were erosion, tissue atrophy, cuff leakage and infection. In another large series, Buzelin and co-workers (personal communication) report a 95% success rate in 80 of 96 patients with the sphincter still in place after a median follow up of 27 months. In this series, 9% of the sphincters were removed, mostly because of erosion. The revision rate was 18%. The series of Mundy et al.[5] and our own series confirm that there is an extremely high risk of complications in patients who have previously received radiotherapy or undergone sling procedures for stress urinary incontinence.

Author	n	Median follow-up years	Success rate	Revision or repair	Erosion/ infusion revision rate
Diokno [6]	32	2.5	91%	21%	0
Mundy* [5]					
A	17	?	15	2	1
B	12	?	4	–	8
Webster [7]	25	2.4	>92%	17%	0
Schreiter [8]	86	5.2	86–90%	50%	43/131
Buzelin [9]	96	2.5	82%	17%	9
Own series	7	5.5	4/7	1/7	3/7**

Table 8.4. Results.
*A: Patients without sling surgery or radiotherapy
 B: Patients with previous sling surgery or radiotherapy.
** One previous sling, two previous radiotherapy.

Pregnancy and the artificial urinary sphincter

Fishman et al.[10] have reported their experience with pregnancies in women with AUS. Seven of their patients became pregnant with a functioning AUS. They delivered nine children, five vaginally and four by caesarian section. No complications related to the artificial sphincter occurred and the authors conclude that women with functioning artificial sphincters do not experience an increased risk of complications during pregnancy and child bearing. One of our patients with myelomeningocele gave birth to a child and the vaginal delivery was uneventful.

Conclusions

In non-neurogenic female incontinence, the artificial urinary sphincter should be avoided in patients with previous sling procedures for stress urinary incontinence and in patients previously administered radiotherapy, due to the unacceptably high risk of erosion and infection. Patients with pure sphincteric incompetence and stable bladders with a normal capacity fare extremely well with the artificial urinary sphincter. It must, however, be pointed out to the patient that the artificial urinary sphincter is a mechanical device with a limited long-term function. The revision rate in most series is 30–50% after five years, and if erosion or infection occur, the device must be removed. However, as an alternative to urinary diversion, the AUS will offer a 90% chance of continence and 80% chance of bladder emptying without catheterization in most cases.

Artificial urinary sphincters in the treatment of neurogenic voiding dysfunction

In addition to all their other disabilities, patients with a neurogenic bladder dysfunction will, if this is left untreated, often develop multiple complications of the urinary tract. Vesicourethral reflux, hydronephrosis, urolithiasis, urinary-tract infection and, finally, end-stage renal failure threaten these patients. Many of them suffer from urinary incontinence and also from an inability to empty the bladder. The urinary incontinence leads to an unpleasant odour and often to serious dermatological problems. In the treatment of these patients, the placement of AUS is a tremendous step-forward but several precautions have to be taken in order to achieve a successful outcome.

Characteristics of neurogenic bladders (Table 8.5)

Conventional surgical techniques used to correct incontinence often fail in the case of neurogenic bladders. Thus, urethral lengthening or bladder-neck tubularization have limited use in these patients.

Detrusor abnormalities, i.e. poor compliance or hyperreflexia, are common and must be corrected before an AUS is placed. Treatment of poor compliance with anticholinergic drugs often fails. Bladder augmentation is generally a good solution in these situations. Subsequent to encouraging results sacral root rhizotomies with or without anterior sacral root stimulation have been presented[1,12]. Patients having bladders with an extremely high compliance or patients with areflexic bladders generally require clean intermittent catheterization (CIC) to facilitate bladder emptying. Hyperreflexic bladders can sometimes be controlled with anticholinergic drugs but, even in this situation, bladder augmentation is often necessary. Even if the hyperreflexia is controlled preoperatively with drugs, the condition might deteriorate after sphincter placement and necessitate secondary bladder augmentation or sacral root rhizotomies.

In neurogenic voiding dysfunction, sphincter disturbances are common. Sphincter detrusor dyssynergia has generally been handled by means of sphincterotomy or bladder flap urethroplasty. The developments of the CIC technique has altered this situation so that many patients manage their dyssynergia with this technique. A pure sphincteric incompetence is best managed with an AUS placement. Scarring and strictures in the bladder neck or sphincteric area might need additional surgical procedures and clean intermittent dilatation. Scarring in the bladder neck area is an indication for cuff placement at the bulbar urethra in the male.

A compromised upper tract might be the result of massive vesicourethral reflux or of a highpressure bladder combined with sphincter detrusor dyssynergia. The prevention of damage to the upper urinary tract is a main undertaking in the treatment of patients with neurogenic bladder dysfunctions.

- Conventional surgical techniques often fail
- Detrusor abnormalities common
  - Compliance
  - Hyperreflexia
  - Areflexia

- Sphincter function disturbances common
  - Dyssynergia
  - Incompetence
  - Scarring

- Compromised upper tract

Table 8.5. Characteristics of neurogenic bladders.

The Uppsala experience with AUS in neurogenic bladders

Material

Between 1985 and 1993, 25 patients have been fitted with 27 sphincters. Seventeen were male and eight female and they had a mean age of 23 years (range 13–41 years). Twenty-two cuffs were placed around the bladder neck and three around the bulbar urethra.

Aetiologies of incontinence

As in other neurogenic bladder materials, the majority of patients (15) had myelodysplasia. Six patients, were operated for benign spinal tumours, two patients were posttraumatic and two had congenital anomalies.

Complementary surgical procedures

Fourteen patients underwent bladder augmentation and two patients are on the waiting list for bladder augmentation, since a hyperreflexic bladder has developed after sphincter placement. Ureteric re-implantation was performed in five patients.

Complications

Four patients required revision for mechanical failure. However, a more serious problem was that as many as eight patients developed erosion and/ or infected devices. At our hospital, two patients have developed a perforation of a continent urinary reservoir, in the more than 100 reservoirs performed, and both these perforations occurred in this patient group. In these cases, the diagnosis was difficult since the general surgeon in the emergency room is often unaware of this rare complication. Of the eight patients with sphincter erosion, two have been given a new sphincter.

Of the remaining six patients, one is continent on CIC, two have been treated with continent urinary diversion and two are incontinent and managed with incontinence pads.

Outcome

Sixteen (64%) of the patients are continent and two have well-functioning devices but require bladder augmentation due to hyperreflexic bladders. One patient was not available to follow-up. Thus, after corrective surgery, 76% of the original 25 patients are continent with functioning sphincters and one with intermittent catheterization without a sphincter; this gives a total continence rate of 80%. One of the female patients has had a normal pregnancy with an uncomplicated vaginal delivery.

Work-up of patients before sphincter placement (Table 8.6)

An intravenous pyelography is necessary to evaluate the function of the kidneys, to reveal any dilation of the upper tracts and to reveal scarring from previous infections or reflux. A voiding cystourethrogram is required to reveal reflux, residual urine or diverticula that might need surgical correction.

A complete urodynamic investigation with electromyelography is also indicated. As previously mentioned, poor bladder compliance, possible dyssynergia, hyperreflexia and sphincter incompetence all need to be taken into consideration in order to select the appropriate treatment for these patients.

- Intravenous pyelography
    Scarring
    Dilation
    Function

- Voiding cystourethrogram
    Reflux
    Residual urine
    Diverticula

- Urodynamics – EMG
    Compliance
    Dyssynergia
    Hyperreflexia
    Sphincter incompetence

Table 8.6. Work-up.

Treatment options

In patients with a good bladder capacity without bladder hyperactivity and with a pure sphincteric incompetence, the placement of an AUS is a straightforward procedure.

In patients with hyperreflexic bladders, treatment with anticholinergic drugs is initiated and, if unsuccessful, bladder augmentation is performed. In this situation, sacral root rhizotomies might be an option.

For low-compliant bladders, drug treatment often fails and augmentation or rhizotomies need to be performed.

Clean intermittent catheterization is instigated in patients with areflexic bladders or with highcompliance bladders. CIC is also indicated in most patients with dyssynergia. Dyssynergia can also be treated with external sphincterotomy or stent placement in the male and bladder flap urethroplasty in the female before AUS placement. These procedures are, however, not without complications and the patients are rendered totally incontinent. If, therefore, the artificial sphincter fails, the patient might have a poorer quality of life than prior to surgery.

In patients with reflux, the latter needs surgical correction if the patient has a dilation of the upper tract.

Considerations of sphincter placement

In the planning of treatment for neurogenic bladder patients, the increased risk of erosion and AUS infection must be taken into account. The results concerning continence are better if the cuff can be placed at the bladder neck rather than placed around the bulbar urethra. An increased degree of freedom is afforded by the patient who is mobile and can make his own way to the toilet. The personal characteristics of the patient, especially concerning motivation, manual dexterity and cooperation, are extremely important. To avoid erosion, a low-pressure balloon (60–70 cmH$_2$O) is recommended but the patient should be informed that this pressure range will give a leakage of urine when the abdominal pressure exceeds the cuff pressure.

Follow-up

To evaluate the upper urinary tract IVP is recommended after 3, 6 and 12 months and then yearly. It is essential that the patient is aware of the necessity of the follow-up procedures in order to preserve kidney function in the long run. Urine cultures are, of course, performed as are laboratory tests like creatinine analyses, etc. Urodynamic investigations are reserved for patients with postoperative leakage. In a study by Buzelin et al.,[13] 55% of his MMC patients developed recurrent incontinence due to detrusor impairment. Poor detrusor behaviour could not be predicted by the preoperative urodynamic investigation.

Complications

Recurrent incontinence is a major complication and often depends on the loss of fluid from the system. The most common leakage is from the cuff. Incontinence might also return due to an atrophy of the tissues underlying the cuff. In this situation, the cuff must often be replaced with one of a smaller size. Kinking of tubes is less common with the new AMS 800 devices and pump failures might evolve but are also uncommon. Infection erosion is a major problem and often probably due to a lack of surgical skill, especially during cuff placement. In most cases, the complete device must be removed and later replaced. In rare cases, the removal of only the cuff can be attempted if a clean erosion is suspected.

Results (Table 8.7)

The results from different series of sphincter placement in neurogenic bladder patients are summarized in Table 8.7. As can be seen in the series

Author	n	Median follow-up	Continence good+	Revision+ repair	Erosion/infection	CIC	Upper-tract dilation
Light (1983) [14] AS 791-792 Spinal cord trauma	49	3	35 (71%)	37 (76%)	12		
Light (1983) [15] Children	87	2	83 (95%)	156 (180%)	2	1	
Jakobsen and Hald (1986) [16] AS 721-792	33	6	25 (76%)	23 (70%)	6 (18%)	1	
Aprikian et al. (1992) [17] AS 800	27	1	-	7 (25%)	4 (14%)	2	
Belloni et al. (1992) [18] AS 800	37	4	33 (90)%	19 (51%)			2 (5%)
Mouriquand and Mollard (1992) [19]	39	5	28 (76%)	23 (59%)	8 (21%)	4	6 (15%)
Barrett et al. (1993) [20] AS 800	59	4	47 + (80%)		3 (5%)	22	3 (5%)
Norlén (1994)	25	5	18 (72%)	4 (16%)	8 (32%)	5	

Table 8.7. Results.

from the early 1980s, the revision rate was high. i.e. almost around 100%. In recent series with the AS 800 and low-pressure balloon (60–70 cmH$_2$O), the revision rate has decreased but a substantial number of revisions and erosion infections still occur. However, even in these early series, the results concerning continence were good in most series; the continence rate is between 75 and 95%.

Conclusions

Placement of an artificial urinary sphincter is a major contribution to the treatment of patients with incontinence due to neurogenic bladders. The continence achieved is above 70% and, in many series, rises up to 90%. Additional surgical procedures such as ureteric re-implantations and bladder augmentations are required in the majority of patients. The revision and complication rates are quite high and should be regarded as part of AUS treatment. Patient compliance during the follow-up period is essential for a good long-term result. As an alternative to urinary diversion, the artificial sphincter can offer excellent continence without external devices and without changing the body image of these, often young, patients.

References

1. Scott FB. Use of the artificial sphincer in the treatment of urinary incontinence. Clin Obstet Gynecol 1995; 12(2): 415–29
2. Barrett DM, Parulkar BG, Kramer SA. Experience with AS 800 artificial sphincter in pediatric and young adult patients. Urology 1993; 42(4): 431–6
3. Sand BK, Bowen LW, Panganiban R, Ostergard DR. The low pressure urethra as a factor in failed retropubic urethorpexy. Obstet Gynecol 1987; 69(3): 399–402
4. Barrett DM, Parulkar BG. The artificial sphincter (AS 800). Experience in children and young adults. Urol Clin North Am 1989; 16(1): 119–32
5. Mundy AR. Artificial sphincters. Br J Urol 1991; 67(3): 225–9
6. Diokno AC, Hollander JB, Alderson TP. Artificial urinary sphincter for recurrent female urinary incontinence: indications and results. J Urol 1987; 138: 778–80
7. Webster GD, Perez LM, Khoury JM, Timmons SL. Management of type III stress urinary incontinence using artificial urinary sphincter. Urology 1992; 34(6): 499–503
8. Schreiter F. The artificial sphincter in the female. Abstract No 42, SIU, Sydney, 1994
9. Buzelin JM, Richard F, Bochereau G. AMS 800 artificial urinary sphincter for treating recurrent female stress urinary incontinence. Personal communication
10. Fishman IJ, Scott FB. Pregnancy in patients with the artificial urinary sphincter. J Urol 1993; 150: 340–1
11. Brindley GS, Polkey CE, Rushton DN, Cardozo L. Sacral anterior root stimulations for bladder control in paraplegia; the first 50 cases. J Neurol Neurosurg Psychiat 1986; 49:1104
12. Koldewijn EL, v. Kerrebrocech PEV, Rosier PFWM et al. Bladder compliance after posterior sacral root rhizotomies and anterior sacral root stimulation. J Urol 1994; 151:955–60
13. Buzelin JM, Richard F, Bochereau G. Impairment of bladder compliance following implantation of artificial urinary sphincter for congenital neuropathic bladder. Personal communications
14. Light JK, Scott FB. Use of the artificial urinary sphincter in spinal cord injury patients. J Urol 1983; 130: 1127–9
15. Light JK, Hawila M, Scott FB. Treatment of urinary incontinence in children: the artificial sphincter versus other methods. J Urol 1983; 130: 518–21

16. Jakobsen H, Hald T. Management of neurogenic urinary incontinence with AMS artificial urinary sphincter. Scand J Urol Nephrol 1986; 20(2): 137–41
17. Aprikian A, Berardinucci G, Pike J, Kiruluta G. Experience with the AS-800 artificial urinary sphincter in myelodysplastic children. Can J Surg 1992; 35(4): 396–400
18. Belloli G, Campobasso P, Mercurella A. Neuropathic urinary incontinence in pediatric patients: management with artificial sphincter. J Ped Surg 1992; 27(11): 1461–4
19. Mouriquand PD, Mollard P. Management of urinary incontinence in neurogenic bladder. Scand J Urol Nephrol 1993; Suppl 141: 28–36

9

Penile implants: history, indications and results of penile implants (mechanical and inflatable)

G. Williams

History

In 1936, Bogoras[1] used a tailored section of ridged cartilage in a similar fashion to the os penis of animals to produce penile rigidity in a reconstructed penis. These grafts were unsatisfactory because of reabsorption, extrusion and infection. Similar findings were reported in 1948 by Bergman et al.[2] Synthetic materials (acrylic splints) implanted beneath Buck's fascia were first used in 1952 by Goodwin and Scott[3,4] and in the 1960s by Loeffler and Sayegh.[5] Beheri was the first to insert a prosthesis within the corpora cavernosa. Though this technique significantly reduced erosion rates,[6,7] the device was poorly tolerated and an incidence of infection and erosion was not eliminated. The silicone implant was first used for the treatment of impotence in 1968.[8] In 1972 Pearman[9] reported the successful use of a silicone silastic prosthetic rod in 126 patients. These were again placed beneath Buck's fascia and, due to a lack of stability, were associated with high extrusion rates and significant discomfort.

The new era of penile implants began in 1973 when Scott et al.[10] introduced the first inflatable penile prosthesis and Small et al.[11] described paired semi-rigid intracorporeal sponge-filled silicone implants.

The inflatable prosthesis described by Scott et al. resulted in a more physiological erection and the penis had a normal size and shape in the flaccid position. The implant was constructed in three parts consisting of two inflatable cylinders, a reservoir and initially two pumps in the scrotum but this was then changed to one. Though attempts have been made to reduce the number of components resulting in a one piece and two piece design, time has shown that these are less than satisfactory. A full circle has evolved, the current three-piece prosthesis manufactured by AMS (American Medical Systems) and MENTOR, direct descendants of the original Scott prosthesis, are the inflatable prostheses of choice.

The non-inflatable prosthesis invented by Small has become the most widely implanted prosthesis ever developed. The Flexi-rod prosthesis introduced in 1977[12] is a semi-rigid rod implant with a softer hinge section beneath the pubis providing better concealment. The first malleable device was introduced by Jonas and Jacobi in 1980.[13] This silicone implant had a twisted silver wire core which increased rigidity and allowed the prosthesis to be bent in any direction. A variety of semi-rigid prostheses have subsequently been developed.

Indications

The penile implant is intended to provide rigidity to the penis upon demand and is indicated in subjects who have lost the ability to produce or maintain an erection sufficient for penetration. They are usually implanted for reasons related to quality of life rather than medical reasons. They have been used to treat impotence resulting from diabetes, spinal cord injury, pelvic surgery, postpriapism, Peyronie's disease, vascular disease and trauma. They have also been implanted in men with psychological impotence. Implantation of a penile prosthesis can help to alleviate feelings of inadequacy in men with erectile dysfunction thereby improving their quality of life.[14,15] There is also a positive impact on the partners of males who have received penile implants and on the relationship as a whole.

The NIH Consensus Conference, December 1992,[18] recommends that the treatment of patients with erectile dysfunction should be individualized and the treatment should be staged with less invasive treatment such as pharmacotherapy, vacuum devices and intracavernosal injections being used first. Penile prostheses should be reserved for patients who fail or refuse other forms of treatment. Possible indications for a penile prosthesis after full discussion with the patient and his partner are shown in Table 9.1.

- Patients who decline alternatives
- Patients who fail alternatives
- Patients who are inappropriate for vascular surgery
- Sickle-cell disease
- Previous priapism
- Coagulopathy

Table 9.1. Indications for a penile prosthesis

Results

In the United States it is estimated that over 500 million US$ are spent annually on new patients undergoing penile prosthesis surgery. Despite this considerable expenditure it was recently reported by the Federal Drug Administration that, though there is reasonable knowledge of the risks and benefits associated with penile prostheses, there is insufficient valid scientific evidence to permit the FDA to perform a risk–benefit analysis.[19] Though widely used since the early 1970s, many prostheses have been subsequently withdrawn from the market. Data on the long-term safety and effectiveness of the currently available implants are limited. The incidences of infection, pain, haematoma, ulceration, migration, extrusion and erosion are often not stated and for the inflatable prosthesis, the incidences of cylinder rupture, leakage, aneurysm, problems with the tubing, valve and reservoir are often unreported. The device is either modified or removed from the market.

Prosthesis selection

Most patients use an inflatable penile prosthesis because of a desire for a more naturally appearing flaccid penis and an increase in penile girth during erection. The number of patients choosing a malleable prosthesis has declined but may be appropriate in patients with limited manual dexterity, severe corporeal fibrosis and those concerned with mechanical dysfunction and the need for further surgery. A non-hydraulic prosthesis is also considerably less expensive.

Results of non-hydraulic prostheses

The AMS malleable 600 prosthesis

This is a paired silicone device with a malleable core of twisted stainless-steel wires wrapped in a synthetic fabric. The diameter of this device is 13 mm; however, by removing the outer silicone jacket this diameter can be changed to 11 mm. The prosthesis comes in three lengths, 12 cm, 15 cm and 20 cm, with 1 cm, 2 cm and 3 cm rear tip extenders. The AMS malleable 600 M has a diameter of 11.5 mm and 9.5 mm and is available in lengths of 12 cm, 14 cm, 16 cm and 18 cm. Experience with this prosthesis had been good[20,21] and mechanical malfunction has not been reported.[22]

Omniphase and Duraphase prostheses (Dacomed)

The Omniphase prosthesis was introduced in 1986 and replaced in September 1987 by the Duraphase. The Duraphase consists of curved cylinders composed of articulating plastic polysulfone balls and sockets. These are larger than those in the Omniphase and create better bendability. A stainless-steel cable runs through the centre of the articulating balls and sockets and is attached at each end to a stainless-steel spring which is fastened to the end of the cylinder body. The cylinder is covered by a polytetrafluoroethylene and silicone sleeve. The cylinder length is 13 cm and has distal tips ranging from 1 to 9 cm and proximal tips from 2 to 9 cm. Only the proximal tips can be trimmed. The prosthesis is supplied in two widths, 10 mm and 12 mm. Since its introduction, the central cable has been reinforced, following four incidences of cable breakages in 63 patients.[23] Of 57 patients in this series, 55 were pleased with the results after four months. The new prosthesis is known as Dura II.

The Finney prosthesis (Surgitek)

This is the only hinged semi-rigid rod. The most recent device is known as the Flexi-Rod II. The rod is made from one piece of soft silicone with an inner, more rigid, silicone material in the distal one-third. The distal end is tapered to fit more precisely underneath the glans. There is a less-rigid 5-cm segment positioned at the penile base to allow the prosthesis to hinge. It is available in diameters of 9 mm, 10.5 mm and 12 mm and in seven lengths, 21.5–29.5 cm. The proximal portion of the device can be trimmed in 0.5 cm trimmable lengths. Finney[24] reported that the vast majority of patients were satisfied with their prosthesis with a removal rate of less than 1%. However, in a patient–partner satisfaction study of 50 men with advanced Peyronie's disease associated with erectile dysfunction and treated with the Finney prosthesis, 48 patients and 29 partners were reassessed with a follow-up of at least 60 months. Only 23 patients and 12 partners were totally satisfied. Amongst the dissatisfied patients (52%), a pencil-like penis, decreasing penile sensitivity, poor concealment and persistent penile deviation were the major complaints. Of the partners, 60% were dissatisfied due to poor penile girth, sensation of a cold glans penis, sensation of unnatural intercourse and dyspareunia. The poor results are not only a reflection on the use of semi-rigid penile prostheses but also an absence of treatment for the Peyronie's disease.[25]

The Jonas prosthesis (BARD)

The original prosthesis was the first malleable rod prosthesis available. It was made of an outer silicone shell with 10 silver wires twisted around each other and embedded in a silicone rubber core. The prosthesis is available in three diameters, 9.5 mm, 11 mm and 13 mm, and to enhance malleability of the two wire rods the middle one-third of the prosthesis is made of a softer silicone material. The soft silicone end of the prosthesis can be cut to produce a prosthesis of the desired length. One hundred patients who had undergone implantation of a Jonas malleable prosthesis were reviewed with a mean follow-up of 30 months.[26] The long-term satisfaction rate was 84% and the probability of having a device without mechanical failure at 23.6 months was estimated to be 96.1%. Thereafter, no additional mechanical failures occurred up to a maximum of 44 months.

The Small–Carrion prosthesis (Mentor)

This prosthesis is available in three diameters, 9 mm, 11 mm and 13 mm. The 9- and 13-mm rods come in five lengths, 12–17 cm and 17–21 cm. The 11-mm rod comes in six lengths from 12 to 18 cm. In a series of 900 patients the author reports that the results have been almost uniformly excellent.[27] There were complications, 53 of which were early and 20 late. Major complications occurred in 57 and minor in 16. The author reports an infection rate of 0.5% as a result of rigorous antibiotic coverage pre- and perioperatively.

Mentor malleable prosthesis

This consists of a silicone rod with an inner double-coiled silver wire wrapped in a Teflon sheath. The rods are trimmable and are available in 9.5 mm, 11 mm and 13 mm diameters. A silicone cap is applied to the trimmed portion. Though one of the most widely used malleable prostheses, there does not appear to be any publications on the effectiveness or long-term benefits of this prosthesis.

Acu-Form (Mentor)

This is a semi-rigid rod prosthesis which contains no internal parts. It is trimmable, comes in the same diameter as the semi-malleable prosthesis and has the same size tail caps. This prosthesis has been in use for three years. As yet, there are no long-term published results on its use.

Hydraulic prostheses

One piece

Following removal from the market in September 1991 of the Surgitek models, Flexiflate II and Uniflate 1000, the only remaining prostheses available are the Hydroflex and the more recently introduced Dynaflex, both manufactured by American Medical Systems. The Dynaflex penile prosthesis is a paired hydraulic device implanted into the corpora cavernosa. The pump is in the distal portion and the reservoir in the proximal portion. The pump transfers fluid from the rear reservoir into a central, non-distensible chamber. When penile rigidity is no longer required the patient bends the penis and maintains the penis in the bent state for approximately 10 s. After release of the penis, fluid leaves the central chamber and returns to the rear tip reservoir. Deflation of the Hydroflex prosthesis is performed by pressure on a release valve just proximal to the pump portion of the prosthesis. Because these devices are self-contained, only a small amount of fluid is transferred between the inflated and deflated states. The deflation flaccidity is not as marked compared to two- or three-piece inflatable prostheses. The Dynaflex is supplied in two diameters, 11 mm and 13 mm; the 11-mm device is available in three lengths, 14 cm, 16 cm and 18 cm, and the 13-mm device in four lengths, 16 cm, 18 cm, 20 cm and 22 cm. The length can be adjusted by the addition of one or more rear tip extenders.

Because of the small size of the pump and its location behind the glans, the Hydroflex prosthesis is probably the most difficult to inflate and deflate and the Dynaflex is difficult to inflate. Patients with poor manual dexterity or neurological impairment involving the hands, may have difficulty with these devices. Elderly patients seem to have difficulty irrespective of whether they have any manual impairment. These prostheses have an inherent rigidity and are not suitable in a very narrow penis as a semi-erection would be present almost all the time. They are also not suitable for patients with a broad penis, i.e. one which can be dilated to size 15 Hegar and beyond as the device will not fill the corpora cavernosum. They are also not suitable in patients who have had a previous multi-component inflatable prosthesis as the one-piece device will not completely fill the cavity. Similarly, in patients with fibrotic corpora from previous infection, erosion or priapism it may be difficult to dilate the corporeal body adequately. If there is a very tight fit, a semi-erect state would be present most of the time.

Because of their inherent rigidity, the penis stretches with lengthening of the intracorporeal measurement and widening of the girth. As a result, the erection becomes inadequate and a high rate of patient dissatisfaction ensues. This is most marked with the 11-mm device.[28] It has been suggested that the ideal candidates for these prostheses are men with slightly narrower than average penises, corporal bodies which easily dilate to size 12 Hegar, and have good finger coordination. In addition, they desire alternate flaccidity and rigidity of the penis and wish to avoid the complexity of a prosthesis with parts outside the corpora cavernosum. The patient also must be satisfied with an erection which does not buckle during penetration nor has pipe-like rigidity.[29] It has been suggested by Wilson[28] that the penile stretching resulting from the insertion of this type of prosthesis is useful in the patient who has developed a large prepubic fat pad with resulting penile recession.

Two piece

The Mentor GFS and Mark II are the only two two-piece devices currently available. The Mark II does not use connectors and the pump reservoir is made of a material less likely to form a capsule. The prostheses are supplied in two versions, one with longer tubing for implantation via the infrapubic approach and one with shorter tubing for implantation via the scrotal approach. Each version comes with cylinders in six lengths, 12–22 cm. Rear tip extenders are available for length adjustment.

Results

Mentor GFS

Early results on 56 patients have been reported.[30] Complications included a scrotal abscess, connector separation in seven and leaking tubing in two. Some patients complained of low volume, particularly when the 20-cc pump was used. In a further study, 12 of 27 two-piece prostheses were revised in a four-year follow-up. Ten revisions resulted from patient dissatisfaction.[28]

GFS Mark II

138 patients were treated with implants over a three-year period with a follow-up of 12–50 months (mean 31.7 months); 93% of the patients and 98% of the partners reported satisfaction with the use of the prosthesis. There was only one mechanical problem involving tubing. Seven implants had to be removed as a result of infection. Thirteen patients required the addition of normal saline through the pump to increase the volume.[31] Similar patient satisfaction has not been reported by Wilson[28] who claims that the penis undergoes stretching and that the 15-cc scrotal reservoir is unable to create an adequate erection. He no longer uses a two-piece prosthesis as a first-line therapy except in patients with extensive abdominal scarring or a history of radiation therapy.

Three piece

American Medical Systems manufacture three, three-piece prostheses: the CX, the Ultrex and the Ultrex plus. These are all direct descendants of the original AMS 700 prosthesis invented by Scott in 1973.

The AMS CX

The cylinders consist of three layers, an outer covering of silicone which prevents tissue ingrowth and provides protection for the middle layer consisting of an expandable woven fabric which provides controlled cylinder girth expansion. The inner layer is a silicone tube into which fluid is pumped, causing it to expand against the controlled expansion of the woven fabric middle layer. The cylinders have a diameter of 12 mm deflated and 18 mm when inflated. The reservoir contains 65 cc and cylinder lengths of 12 cm, 15 cm, 18 cm and 21 cm are available with 1 cm, 2 cm 3 cm rear tip extenders. A smaller version of this device, the AMS 700 CXM, is available. The reservoir is 50 cc and four cylinders 12 cm, 14 cm, 16 cm and 18 cm with a diameter of 9.5 mm when deflated and 14.2 mm when inflated are available.

To date, no cylinder aneurysms have been reported and the low incidence of tubing leaks at the level of the connector has been reduced further by using straight quick-connect connectors rather than curved suture tie connectors. Furlow and Motley[32] reported on 63 patients, the majority of whom were undergoing revisional surgery, 35 with aneurysmal dilatation. In a three-year follow-up, there was no recurrence of the primary disorder that necessitated revision; cylinder leakage occurred in only one patient and erosion necessitating cylinder removal in two. A longer follow-up of these patients with an additional 31 patients has been subsequently reported with similar results.[33] In a review of 214 patients treated with this device with a mean follow-up of 56 months, life-table analysis to calculate the probability of the cylinder and device as a whole surviving six years was 97% for the cylinder and 90% for the device as a whole. The incidence of cylinder leak was 0.7%.[34]

The AMS Ultrex

This is a modification of the CX cylinder. The middle fabric layer provides controlled girth expansion allowing the cylinder diameters to vary between 12 mm deflated and 18 mm inflated. Unlike the CX cylinder, the Ultrex permits controlled length expansion of at least 20%. There are four cylinder lengths, 12 cm, 15 cm, 18 cm and 21 cm, and 1 cm, 2 cm and 3 cm rear tip extenders. There is a 65 cc and 100 cc reservoir.

In a report concerning length expansion of this device, the intraoperative pubis to mid glans length increased from the deflated to the inflated state from 1 to 4 cm with a mean of 1.9 cm.[35] However, to actually cause penile lengthening, the patient must be highly motivated and keep the device pumped up for several hours each day. Experience with this prosthesis is limited. In a series of 100 patients with a follow-up of 2–34 months (mean 14 months) there were two mechanical failures, one a reservoir leak and the other a pump leak, and one device was explanted because of infection.[36]

The Ultrex Plus

This has only been recently introduced and is supplied with a prefilled pump, and cylinders which are connected directly to the pump. The reservoir is separate and is implanted empty and filled after implantation. There is therefore only one component that needs to be filled at operation and only one tubing connection needs to be made. The results of clinical trials are awaited.

Mentor

The original Mentor inflatable three-piece prosthesis was introduced in 1984. This was superseded in 1990 by the Mentor Alpha 1. This inflatable prosthesis must be considered the current prosthesis of choice. The cylinder is constructed of Bioflex, a polyurethane polymer. The pump is pre-attached to the cylinders which eliminates two of the three connectors and has only a straight connector between the pump and reservoir. There are six cylinder lengths, 12 cm, 14 cm, 16 cm, 18 cm, 20 cm and 22 cm, with rear tip extenders of 1 cm, 2 cm and 3 cm. There are three reservoir sizes of

60 cc, 75 cc and 100 cc. The device comes with long tubing lengths for infrapubic implantation and shorter tubing lengths for scrotal implantation. This prosthesis carries a life-time warrant.

In a series of 193 implants using one straight connector, only five were revised for mechanical failure in a two-year period.[28] In a series of 333 patients followed for an average of 15.4 months, there were 25 complications with 15 who required re-operation. Nine of these were due to a split in the exit tubing from the pump which has resulted in the manufacturers reinforcing the exit tubing. Of note, only four patients were admitted for more than 24 hours for their surgery.[37] In a further study of 50 patients, data were obtained from medical records and patient completed structured questionnaires: 98% of the patients and 96% of the partners were satisfied with the device; all were satisfied with the girth and rigidity but only 92% were satisfied with the length; 98% said they would undergo the procedure again and would recommend the implant to other impotent patients.[38]

Penile implants for specific conditions

Peyronie's disease
Controlled expansion cylinders have been shown to be particularly effective when implanted into patients with known penile curvature secondary to Peyronie's disease. The intrinsic design of these cylinders resists the tendency of the erect penis to bend. As a result, the need for an additional penile-straightening procedure either with relaxing incisions, Nesbit's procedure or the insertion of a corporeal graft becomes unnecessary. If relaxing incisions are required these cylinders do not herniate through the defect in the tunica. Good results have also been reported in patients treated with a semi-rigid or malleable rod penile prosthesis.[27,39]

Spinal cord injury
There has been a gradual reduction in the use of penile implants in patients with spinal cord injury. This is due both to the frequency of complications and the efficacy of drug-induced erections or vacuum erection devices. Spinal cord injury patients have been reported to be at increased risk of infection of the prosthesis. An incidence as high as 15% has been reported.[40] Such patients are also at increased risk from erosion, in part because of infection but also due to lack of sensation. An inflatable prosthesis is to be preferred. In a series of 18 patients[41] using old-style inflatable penile prostheses, the incidence of primary infection was 5.5%. The revision rate was 44.3% but most of these were due to mechanical failures in these early inflatable prostheses. One patient developed urethral

erosion secondary to a catheter injury. Steidle and Mulcahy have recommended a perineal urethrotomy or suprapubic catheter in spinal cord injury patients treated with a semi-rigid prosthesis in view of the high rate of erosion in patients using intermittent self-catheterization.[42]

Priapism

Initial reports suggested that patients with corporeal fibrosis as a result of sickle-cell disease, intracavernosal injection therapy or following removal of an infected implant were best treated with a semi-rigid prosthesis since the inflatable prosthesis may not overcome corporeal rigidity.[43] However, by using techniques such as plaque incision or excision and reconstruction with a Dacron or polytetrafluoroethylene patch, an inflatable prosthesis can usually be inserted.[44]

Complications of penile prostheses

Infection

This is one of the most serious potential complications of implantation and may cause significant patient morbidity.[45,46] The presence of infection usually requires the removal of the device and may result in the inability to replace a new device due to corporeal fibrosis.[47] The infection may lead to gangrene and extensive tissue loss.[48] The overall incidence of infection has been estimated to be around 2% with 0.6–16.7% for non-hydraulic devices, 3–8.1% for one-piece hydraulic devices and 0.8–8% for three-piece hydraulic devices.[49] Implantation to new diabetics has an infection risk of around 3% which rises to 21% in a diabetic undergoing a revisionary procedure (Fig. 9.1). By defining strict protocols for implantation of penile prostheses, a significant reduction in the loss of implants following penile prosthetic surgery has been reported.[50] There is a life-long risk of late haematogenous spread of infection from distant sources.[51] Patients with a penile implant require antibacterial prophylaxis for any subsequent dental or surgical procedure.

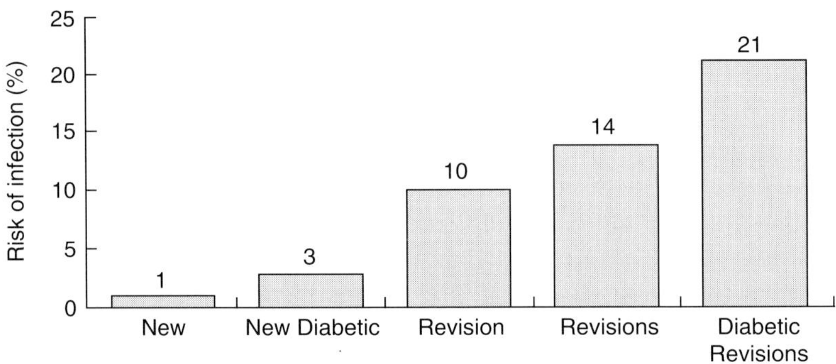

Fig. 9.1. Penile implants: infection risk.

Migration and extrusion

Migration is the movement of the penile implant within the body and extrusion is where the implant occupies an abnormal external position. Extrusion is usually associated with wound dehiscence at the incision site but proximal migration has also been reported. Migration of the reservoir intra-abdominally, movement of the pump to mid-scrotum and movement of the cylinder to the site of perforation posteriorly into the buttocks or from one corpus to the other have all been reported.

Erosion

Erosion is the destruction of tissue and usually occurs distally through the urethra or the glans penis. It has also been reported to occur through bowel, bladder and ileal conduits by the reservoir and through the scrotal wall by the pump. It is often associated with infection but ischaemia secondary to athero-sclerosis, diabetes or too large a prosthesis also plays a role. It is more likely to occur in patients who suffer from lack of sensation or require urethral catheter-ization. Though erosion usually requires removal of the device, Furlow and Goldwasser[52] were able to successfully salvage 16 of 22 cases of scrotal pump erosion, 8 of 8 cases of reservoir erosion but none of 2 cases of cylinder erosion.

Mechanical failure

Long-term results of the new inflatable penile prostheses are not available but early reports of the AMS Ultrex Plus and the Mentor Alpha 1 which require only one sutureless connector suggests that a mechanical failure rate of less than 3% can be achieved. With these improvements in design, the recipients of penile inflatable implants can be expected to exhibit a high degree of satisfaction with regard to sexual function and overall quality of life.[53,54]

Summary

Most of the current literature relates to prostheses which are no longer marketed. With improvements in pharmacotherapy given not only intracavernosally but also urethrally and orally, and with better and more specific vasodilating and smooth-muscle relaxing agents, the insertion of a penile prosthesis will take on a much smaller role. The long-term safety and effectiveness of new devices is needed. In particular, we need to be able to identify the subgroups of the population in whom the benefits of implantation outweigh the attendant risks. The pre-operative work-up needs to be standardized as does the management following implantation to reduce the risks of infection. There are too few studies in patient and partner satisfaction. In the longer term, the potential risks associated with silicone particle shedding, silicone gel leaking and the long-term effects of degradation of polyurethane elastomer are not understood.

References

1. Bogoras NA. Über die volle plastische Wiederherstellung eines rum koitus fahigen penis (Peniplastica totalis). Zentralbl Chir 1936; 63: 1271–4
2. Bergman RT, Howard AH, Barnes RW. Plastic reconstruction of the penis. J Urol 1948; 59: 1174–82
3. Goodwin WE, Scott WW. Phalloplasty. J Urol 1952; 68: 903–8
4. Goodwin WE, Scardino PL, Scott WW. Penile prosthesis for impotence: case report. J Urol 1981; 126: 409
5. Loeffler RA, Sayegh ES. Perforated acrylic implants in management of organic impotence. J Urol 1960; 84: 559–61
6. Beheri GE. The problem of impotence solved by a new surgical operation. Kasr el Aini J Surg 1960; 1: 390–4
7. Beheri GE. Surgical treatment of impotence. Plast Reconstr Surg 1966; 38: 92–7
8. Lash H. Silicone implant for impotence. J Urol 1968; 100: 709–10
9. Pearman RO. Insertion of a silastic penile prosthesis for the treatment of organic sexual impotence. J Urol 1972; 107: 802–6
10. Scott FB, Bradley WE, Timm GW. Management of erectile impotence: use of implantable inflatable prosthesis. Urology 1973; 2: 80–2
11. Small MP, Carrion HM, Gordon JA. Small–Carrion penile prothesis: a new implant for management of impotence. Urology 1975; 5: 479–86
12. Finney RP. New hinged silicone implant. J Urol 1977; 118: 585–7
13. Jonas U, Jacobi GH. Silicone–silver penile prosthesis: description, operative approach and results. J Urol 1980; 123: 865–7
14. Beaser RA, Van der Hoel C, Jacobsen AM et al. Experience with penile prostheses in the treatment of impotence in diabetic men. JAMA 1982; 248: 943–8
15. Tiefer L, Moss S, Melman A. Follow-up of patients and partners experiencing penile prosthesis malfunction and corrective surgery. J Sex Marital Therapy 1991; 17: 113–28
16. Pedersen B, Tiefer L, Ruiz M, Melman A. Evaluation of patients and partners 1 to 4 years after penile prosthesis surgery. J Urol 1988; 139: 956–8
17. Tiefer L, Pedersen B, Melman A. Psychosocial follow-up of penile prosthesis implant patients and partners., J Sex Marital Therapy 1988; 14: 184–201
18. NIH Consensus Statement: Impotence. Vol 10, No. 4, December 7–9 1992
19. Department of Health and Human Services Food and Drug Administration. Gastro-enterology–Urology devices. Federal Register, Part II, 1993, Vol 58, No. 80, pp. 25906
20. Dorflinger T, Bruskewitz R. AMS malleable penile prosthesis. Urology 1986; 28: 480–5
21. Moul JW, McLeod DG. Experience with the AMS 600 malleable penile prosthesis. J Urol 1986; 135: 929–31
22. Nielsen KT, Bruskewitz RC. Semi-rigid and malleable rod penile prostheses. Urol Clin N Am 1989; 16: 13–23
23. Mulcahy JJ, Krane RJ, Lloyd LK et al. Duraphase penile prosthesis results of clinical trials in 63 patients. J Urol 1990; 143: 518–19
24. Finney RP. Finney-Flexi rod prosthesis. Urology 1984; 23: 79–82
25. Montorsi F, Guazzoni G, Bergamaschi F, Rigatti P. Patient–partner satisfaction with semi-rigid penile prostheses for Peyronie's disease: a 5-year follow up study. J Urol 1993; 150: 1819–21
26. Benson RC Jr, Patterson DE, Barrett DM. Long term results with the Jonas malleable penile prosthesis. J Urol 1985; 134: 899–901
27. Small MP. Surgical treatment of impotence with Small–Carrion prosthesis. Urology 1984; 23: 93–7
28. Wilson SK. Current treatment of impotence with inflatable penile prosthesis examined. AUA Today, September 1992
29. Mulcahy JJ. The Hydroflex self-contained inflatable prosthesis: experience with 100 patients. J Urol 1988; 140: 1422–3
30. Engel RME, Fein RL. Mentor GFS inflatable prosthesis. Urology 1990; 35: 405–6
31. Fein RL. GFS Mark II inflatable penile prosthesis: four-year clinical study. Urology 1994; 43: 209–13
32. Furlow WL, Motley RC. The inflatable penile prosthesis: clinical experience with a new controlled expansion cylinder. J Urol 1988; 139: 945–6

33. Knoll LD, Furlow WL, Motley RC. Clinical experience implanting an inflatable penile prosthesis with controlled expansion cylinder. Urology 1990; 36: 502–4

34. Quesada ET, Light JK. The AMS 700 inflatable penile prosthesis: long term experience with the controlled expansion cylinders. J Urol 1993; 149: 46–8

35. Montague DK, Lakin MM. Early experience with the controlled girth and length expanding cylinder of the AMS Ultrex penile prosthesis. J Urol 1992; 148: 1444–6

36. Montague DK, Lakin MM. Penile prostheses. In Bennett AH (ed) Impotence diagnosis and management of erectile dysfunction. Philadelphia, WB Saunders, 1994; 282

37. Randrup E, Wilson S, Mobley D et al. Clinical experience with Mentor Alpha #1 inflatable penile prosthesis. Urology 1993; 42: 305–8

38. Garber BB. Mentor Alpha #1 inflatable penile prosthesis: patient satisfaction and device reliability. Urology 1994; 43: 214–17

39. Raz S, de Kernion JB, Kaufman JJ. Surgical treatment of Peyronie's disease: a new approach. J Urol 1977; 117: 598–601

40. Fallon B, Ghanem H. Infected penile prostheses: incidence and outcomes. Int J Impotence Res 1989; 1: 175–7

41. Light JK, Scott FB. Management of neurogenic impotence with inflatable penile prosthesis. Urology 1981; 17: 341–3

42. Steidle CP, Mulcahy JJ. Erosion of penile prostheses: a complication of urethral catheterisation. J Urol 1989; 142: 736–9

43. Bertram RA, Carson CC, Webster GD. Implantation of penile prostheses in patients impotent after priapism. Urology 1985; 26: 325–7

44. Fishman IJ. Corporeal reconstruction procedures for complicated penile implants. Urol Clin N Am 1989; 16: 73–90

45. Kabalin JN, Kessler R. Infectious complications of penile prosthesis surgery. J Urol 1988; 139: 953–5

46. Thomalla JV, Thompson ST, Rowland RG, Mulcahy JJ. Infectious complications of penile prosthetic implants. J Urol 1987; 138: 35–47

47. Carson CC. Infections in genito-urinary prostheses. Urol Clin N Am 1989; 16: 139–47

48. McClellan DS, Masih BK. Grangrene of the penis as a complication of penile prosthesis. J Urol 1985; 133: 862–3

49. Moul JW, Carson CC. Infectious complications of penile prostheses. Infect Urol 1989; 97–102

50. Lynch MJ, Scott GM, Inglis JA, Pryor JP. Reducing the loss of implants following penile prosthesis surgery. Br J Urol 1994; 73: 423–7

51. Carson CC, Robertson CN. Late haematogenous infection of penile prostheses. J Urol 1988; 139: 50–2

52. Furlow WL, Goldwasser B. Salvage of the eroded inflatable penile prosthesis: a new concept. J Urol 1987; 138: 312–14

53. McLaren RH, Barrett DM. Patient and partner satisfaction with the AMS 700 penile prosthesis. J Urol 1992; 147: 62–5

54. Whalen RK, Merrill DC. Patient satisfaction with the Mentor inflatable penile prosthesis. Urology 1991; 37: 531–9

Artificial bladder replacement

10

D. M. Barrett   D. C. O'Sullivan
B. G. Parulkar   M. G. Donovan

Introduction

Carcinoma of the bladder is one of the most common genitourinary malignancies. The incidence of carcinoma of the bladder in the United States in 1990 was 49 000 cases.[1] Total cystectomy is the best treatment in about 5000 to 8000 of these patients. Another 3000–4000 cystectomies plus innumerable urinary diversions are undertaken every year for disabling benign bladder disease which may be congenital (ectopic viscera, neurogenic bladder) or acquired (interstitial cystitis, chronic infection such as tuberculosis, and radiation).[2] Most of these urinary diversions are undertaken using segments of intestine for conduit or reservoir replacement. These conduits may exit the anterior abdominal wall or may in fact be attached to the urethra so that the urine can be passed through the normal channel.

Although these intestinal urinary diversions are considerably better than bringing the ureters themselves to the skin, the numerous physical and psychological complications associated with their use has spurred investigation into total alloplastic replacement of the lower urinary tract. With this approach, however, many setbacks have occurred. The main problems that must be overcome are hydronephrosis and infection from urinary stasis, and encrustation of the luminal surface of the prosthesis.[3]

The ideal prosthetic bladder would have the following characteristics:[4]

- allowance for variation in volume storage, low-pressure filling and storage, and low-pressure voiding without reflux into the renal units;
- have a mechanism for volitional control and voiding;
- be able to reduce the operating time involved in creating a new conduit and have no metabolic complications;
- ideally, be available to every patient regardless of their general condition, age and sex, and would not use any portion of the patient's intestine for its function;
- be made of a totally inert material which is non-carcinogenic, biocompatible and non-degradable.

From a surgical standpoint, a prosthetic bladder would be easy to implant and be accessible for repairs and replacements if needed. The most important factor would be its ability to preserve and protect the function of the kidneys and maintain renal function for an intermediate time into the future. Overall, it would enhance the patient's quality of life and protect life expectancy.

Mayo artificial bladder design

For the last 15 years we have pursued the challenge of developing an artificial bladder. Initial efforts concentrated on developing materials that were biocompatible and did not allow for encrustation and stone formation.[5] Subsequently, work was undertaken to develop the ideal method of connecting the ureters and the urethra to a prosthetic bladder. Next, a storage prototype was developed with a continence mechanism.[4]

Currently, we have developed a concept that has, in laboratory animals, proved to be efficacious at least over the intermediate term. This artificial bladder concept was granted a United States patent on December 6 1994 (patent number 5370690)[6] (Fig. 10.1).

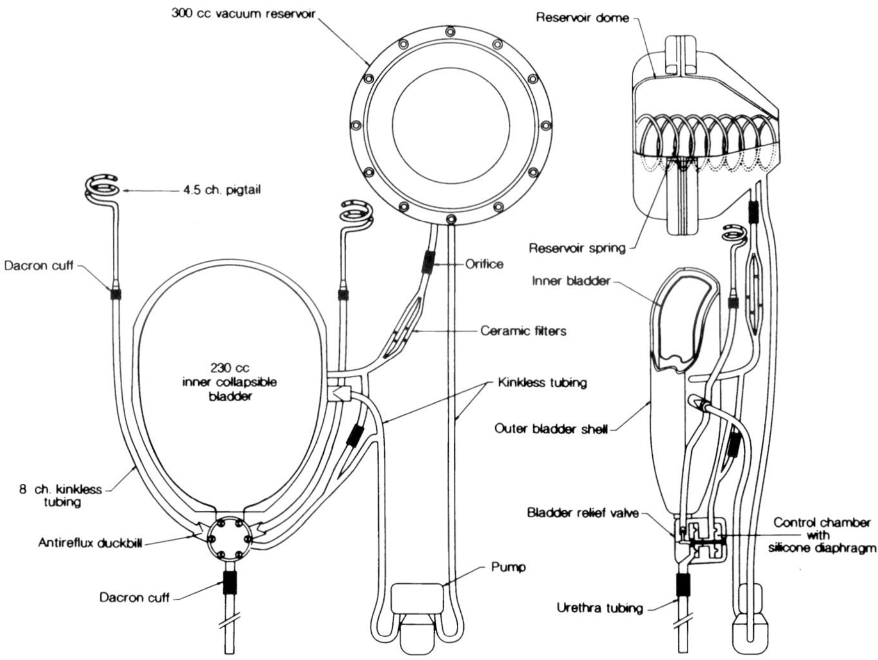

Fig. 10.1. Anterior and lateral views of artificial complete bladder system.

Material

Ureter

The ureter is made of 8 F silicone tubing reinforced with a nylon spiral to prevent kinking. At its proximal end is a 4.5 F Silitek pigtail for insertion into the renal pelvis, and a 0.5-cm Dacron cuff facilitates anastomosis with the ureteric stump. At its distal end the ureter is attached to a polysulfone housing that contains a silicone latex rubber duckbill antireflux valve. This unit is attached to the urethral valve unit.

Bladder

The artificial bladder is constructed of two shells – a 230-ml flexible silicone inner bladder and a 300-ml rigid polysulfone outer shell. These two shells are connected only at the bladder neck, and an 80-ml space intervenes. The outer shell has two connectors: (1) an inlet from the pump, which has an antireflux valve, and (2) an outlet to the reservoir.

Reservoir

The reservoir has a rigid polysulfone base, shaped like a truncated cone, and a flexible silicone dome, which are compressed together by two stainless-steel rings. An 11-cm stainless-steel spring inside the reservoir creates negative pressure within the entire system when it is compressed. The reservoir has an inlet that drains saline from the enclosed space in the bladder and an outlet connected to the pump.

Orifices or flow resistors

A polysulfone orifice (Air Logic, Racine, WI) in continuity in the tubing between the bladder and the reservoir regulates the rate of refilling of the reservoir. Three orifices with internal diameters of 0.125, 0.15 and 0.175 mm were tested with this bladder. Four parallel ceramic filters, with 30-μm pores, placed between the bladder and the orifice, remove any particulate matter that might obstruct the orifice.

Urethral valve

The machined polysulfone urethral valve is divided into two main chambers. The first chamber, which is connected to both the urethra and the bladder, acts as the conduit for the urine. Within this chamber is a stainless-steel poppet on one end of the central rod. This poppet has a sharp rim around its edge that abuts the silicone seat to create a water-tight seal that obstructs the flow of urine when closed. The central rod is suspended in two flexible silicone diaphragms and is thus mobile in a to-and-fro motion. The central rod traverses the valve unit to the second chamber or control unit. This chamber is connected to both the reservoir and the pump, so that during the bladder cycle, pressure changes act on the diaphragm and force the central rod back and forth and consequently open or close the valve at the other end. A spring and screw cap on the end of the central rod ensure that the valve is closed in the resting position and also allow the opening, or leak point, pressure to be varied.

The urethra is an 18 F silicone tube with a Dacron cuff at its proximal end for attachment to the urethral stump. The pump is made of silicone, is unidirectional, and has a 2-ml volume.

Methods

The pressure–flow characteristics of each component and of the entire bladder system were tested to determine the pressures generated at various flow rates of urine, with particular reference to the pressures in the ureters.

Ureteric valves and ureters were tested at flow rates of 0–200 ml/h and the valves were examined for reflux. The urethral valve was set up with a saline-filled syringe and a transducer attached to the control chamber and the infusion pump and another transducer connected to the valve inlet. The opening, or leak point, pressure and the pressures generated at flow rates up to 50 ml/min were then measured while pressures varied from +20 cmH$_2$O to −130 cmH$_2$O in the control chamber. Pressures generated in the reservoir during emptying and filling were also measured.

The entire bladder system was tested by attaching the infusion pump and a transducer to the ureters. Another connector was placed in the outer shell of the bladder to measure pressures generated in the enclosed space during the bladder cycle. Pressures inside the silicone bladder could not be measured directly because a transducer could not be placed within its lumen. Pressures in the inner bladder should be similar to those in the ureter during the filling phase. A duckbill valve was added to the urethra to simulate the vaginal tissues and natural urethra that would be present after implantation in the dog.[6]

Discussion

The artificial bladder described here was designed to overcome the major problems encountered with previous bladder designs. The main cause of failure with previous artificial bladders has been the development of hydronephrosis and renal failure. Sometimes the cause has been ureteric obstruction from formation of a papilloma, encrustation and ureteric kinking. The pigtail on the ureter in the current design overcomes the problem of formation of a papilloma because placement in the renal pelvis decreases irritation and this location is distant from the site of anastomosis. The non-kinking silicone tubing minimizes the possibility of the other problems. Development of hydronephrosis and renal failure without apparent obstruction is due to the difficulty with which the ureteric remnant propels urine along an adynamic tube. Hydronephrosis is less of a problem with short ureteric prostheses but is common with long ureteric prostheses and total bladder replacements because the longer the segment replaced, the greater the workload on the remaining ureter.

Normal intrapelvic pressure is $< 10\,\text{cmH}_2\text{O}$, that during the peristaltic wave is approximately $25\,\text{cmH}_2\text{O}$, and bladder pressure is $10\,\text{cmH}_2\text{O}$ throughout most of the filling cycle. Therefore, the normal ureter tends to draw urine out of the renal pelvis and transfer it to the bladder, which actively relaxes. Previously, almost all artificial bladder replacements have relied on ureteric pressure to expand a flexible bladder. In the model described herein, the negative pressure inside the outer shell ensures that no back pressure is on the renal pelvis and thus aims to prevent hydronephrosis. In the design tested, the early ureteric pressure is excessively low but can be regulated somewhat by use of a smaller orifice. We have also developed a negative pressure regulator that is placed between the bladder and the reservoir. It occludes flow when the bladder pressure decreases below $-35\,\text{cmH}_2\text{O}$ and re-opens when the pressure increases to $-30\,\text{cmH}_2\text{O}$. Our goal, however, is to maintain bladder pressure at $-10\,\text{cmH}_2\text{O}$, but at this pressure and with the relatively low flow rates involved, effective functioning of a negative pressure regulator is difficult. Further studies and development are needed.

Apoil and associates designed a bistable bladder that generated a pressure of $-40\,\text{cmH}_2\text{O}$, but hydronephrosis still occurred because expansion was restricted by the development of a fibrous capsule.[7] Lutzeyer and colleagues also developed a negative pressure system that depends on rebound of the bladder wall after emptying.[8] This design worked well in seven sheep for a mean of seven months. These investigators have not reported the pressures generated in the renal pelvis during filling.

In all reported studies in which the bladder has been placed intra-abdominally, a fibrous capsule has developed around the prosthesis and has led to restriction of filling and emptying. The hard outer shell of the current model prevents interference from the surrounding tissues and allows generation of the necessary expulsive force. In most prostheses, gravity has been the basis of bladder emptying. Although this principle has been effective, bench testing has shown that most models have large residual volumes of urine after implantation. Retention is also caused by the fibrous capsule, which inhibits complete collapse of the bladder. Resistance from the urethra and the external sphincter also acts against gravity and prevents complete emptying. Rigotti and co-workers were the first to incorporate effective active emptying into a bladder model, but a percutaneous connection to an air pump was necessary.[9] The model developed by Lutzeyer and associates is emptied by compression of the subcutaneous bladder against the underlying fascia. In our model, the implanted pump ensures complete emptying by generating a pressure of $400\,\text{cmH}_2\text{O}$ within the outer shell. Because of this high pressure, antireflux valves are imperative; without them, any malfunction of the urethral valve would lead to extreme intrapelvic pressures and rupture of the pelvis.

Many prosthetic bladders have had problems with leakage of urine at the urethral anastomosis because the external sphincter and thick vaginal wall were distal to the prosthesis. In the current model the urethra extends beyond the sphincter into the vagina.

The urethral valve used is essential to the effective functioning of the system. It maintains continence during filling and opens completely when the bladder is being emptied; thus, resistance is minimized. The high pressures needed to open the valve when the pressure in the reservoir is low are not of significance *in vivo* because, as the flow of urine increases, the reservoir refills more quickly, up to a rate of 400 ml/h at its greatest negative pressure. This increased filling rate decreases the negative pressure in the control unit and would allow overflow if the output of urine were even greater than this. The maximal back pressure that can occur in the renal pelvis (20 cmH$_2$O at 200 ml/h with a full bladder) is the combined resistance of the ureter, resistance of the ureteric valve and overflow resistance of the urethral valve. For *in vivo* studies in 25-kg dogs, the mean flow rates used are 40–80 ml/h. The tortuous channel through the valve prevents the passage of any monitoring equipment; this drawback will be changed in future models. Also, the machined surfaces could act as a nidus for encrustation and they will be coated with silicone in future.

Conclusion

The new artificial bladder design described in this report addresses many of the problems experienced with previous designs.[6] Its main advance is in the use of negative-pressure drainage of the renal pelves, which should avoid the hydronephrosis that has occurred with most previous models. This is the first prosthetic bladder in which the pressure effects that occur in the kidney have been measured. The risk of infection is minimized by having a completely implantable system, the only external connection being the urethra (which cannot be eliminated). In addition, the risk of encrustation is decreased by having a mainly silicone system that empties completely, leaving no residual urine that could cause infection or formation of stones.

References

1. Boring CC, Squires TS, Tong T. Cancer Statistics (1992) CA-A Cancer J Clin 1992; 42(1): 19–38
2. Catalona WJ. Bladder cancer. In Gillenwater JY, Grayhack JT, Howard SS, Duckett JW (eds) Adult and pediatric urology, Vol. 1. Chicago, IL, Year Book Medical Publishers, 1987; 1000–43
3. Barrett DM, Donovan MG. Prosthetic bladder augmentation and replacement. Sem Urol 1984; 2(3): 167–75
4. Parulkar BG, Barrett DM, Fung E. Designing a model for in vitro testing of urine compatible materials using synthetic urine. Presented at the June 1991 American Urological Association Annual Meeting
5. Donovan MG. The testing of biocompatibility of alloplastic materials in the genitourinary

tract suitable for use as prosthetic materials. Thesis, University of Dublin, Trinity College, Dublin, 1984

6. Barrett DM, O'Sullivan DC, Parulkar BG et al. Artificial bladder replacement: a new design concept. Mayo Clin Proc 1992; 66: 215–20

7. Apoil A, Granger A, Sausse A, Stern A. Experimental and clinical studies of prosthetic bladder replacement. In Wagenknecht LV, Furlow WL, Auvert J (eds) Genitourinary reconstruction with prostheses. Stuttgart, Georg Thieme, 1981; 75–80

8. Lutzeyer W, Gerlach R, Heinrich B, Gregoir W. Development and animal experimental investigation of an artificial bladder with sphincter. Presented at the 95th Annual Meeting of the American Association of Genitourinary Surgeons.

9. Rigotti E, Randone D, Tizzani A et al. Sostituzione totale della vescica con protesi: ricerche sperimentali; primi risultati. Minerva Urol 1976; 28: 1–5

Index